Family-Based Therapy for Latine Adolescents

Family-Based Therapy for Latine Adolescents

The CIFFTA Model

Daniel A. Santisteban
Maite P. Mena
David Santisteban

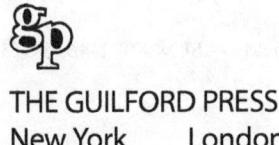

THE GUILFORD PRESS
New York   London

Copyright © 2025 The Guilford Press
A Division of Guilford Publications, Inc.
www.guilford.com

All rights reserved

No part of this book may be reproduced, translated, stored in a retrieval system, or transmitted, in any form or by any means, electronic, mechanical, photocopying, microfilming, recording, or otherwise, without written permission from the publisher.

Printed in the United States of America

This book is printed on acid-free paper.

For product and safety concerns within the EU, please contact GPSR@taylorandfrancis.com, Taylor & Francis Verlag GmbH, Kaufingerstraße 24, 80331 München, Germany.

Last digit is print number: 9 8 7 6 5 4 3 2 1

The authors have checked with sources believed to be reliable in their efforts to provide information that is complete and generally in accord with the standards of practice that are accepted at the time of publication. However, in view of the possibility of human error or changes in behavioral, mental health, or medical sciences, neither the authors, nor the editor and publisher, nor any other party who has been involved in the preparation or publication of this work warrants that the information contained herein is in every respect accurate or complete, and they are not responsible for any errors or omissions or the results obtained from the use of such information. Readers are encouraged to confirm the information contained in this book with other sources.

Library of Congress Cataloging-in-Publication Data is available from the publisher.

ISBN 978-1-4625-5753-0 (paperback) — ISBN 978-1-4625-5754-7 (hardcover)

To my wife, Yoli: Thank you for your unwavering love, wisdom, and support.

To my siblings, Elizabeth, David, and Arturo; my kids, Javier, Francesco, Denise, and Rick; and my grandkids: Thank you for continuing to multiply the blessings in our lives.

To my parents, Maxi and Arturo, who taught us the meaning of love, courage, wisdom, integrity, and sacrifice: We honor and love you.

—Daniel A. Santisteban

Danny, Eric, and Sofia: Your steadfast love and support mean the world to me; thank you for allowing me to pursue my passion.

To my parents: Your courage to start over from nothing taught me the importance of resilience and the strength of family.

Aya: I am incredibly grateful for the lessons you taught me about faith, culture, and perseverance, and for never letting go of my hand.

—Maite P. Mena

To my son, Leonard; my daughter, Alejandra; and my grandchildren. And to my parents and relatives who made the difficult decision to emigrate with their families, and by so doing gave my generation, and generations to come, the opportunity to exercise the right to choose our own paths.

—David Santisteban

About the Authors

Daniel A. Santisteban, PhD, is Cofounder and Director of Research at Training and Implementation Associates and Professor Emeritus at the University of Miami. A researcher in the area of culturally informed adolescent and family therapy since the 1990s, he is the primary developer of Culturally Informed and Flexible Family-Based Treatment for Adolescents (CIFFTA). Dr. Santisteban's current work focuses on creating and testing an evidence-based platform for training, coaching, and implementation that uses clinical simulations. He has authored over 50 articles and chapters and has received career research awards from the American Family Therapy Association, the National Hispanic Science Network, and Division 45 of the American Psychological Association (Society for the Psychological Study of Culture, Ethnicity, and Race).

Maite P. Mena, PsyD, is Research Assistant Professor in the School of Education and Human Development at the University of Miami and the codeveloper of CIFFTA. Her research since the early 2000s has focused on the unique stressors faced by minority populations, such as immigration-related separations, and how CIFFTA can positively influence outcomes. Dr. Mena's current work focuses on evaluating CIFFTA's effectiveness in real-world settings and enhancing CIFFTA's trauma focus and interventions. She is actively involved in providing CIFFTA implementation support and training and coaching clinicians across the country. Dr. Mena has published in peer-reviewed journals and has presented on CIFFTA at national and local conferences.

David Santisteban, PhD, is Cofounder of Training and Implementation Associates, which supports mental health professionals, treatment agencies, and funding agencies in meeting complex implementation challenges. His early work in academic clinical research focused on the development of culturally appropriate prevention and treatment strategies for Hispanic adolescents and their families. Dr. Santisteban served as Co-Principal Investigator and/or Project Director on several clinical research grants, published and presented on the mental health needs of Hispanic families, and consulted to a number of national programs and initiatives. Since transitioning to the private sector, he has focused on the utilization of technology and simulation to develop innovative assessment and training strategies. Dr. Santisteban is currently the Principal Investigator of a National Institute of Mental Health Small Business Innovation Research grant. The aim of the grant is to create training and dissemination innovations using state-of-the-art technology (e.g., avatars, digital voices) and clinical simulations.

Preface

We are grateful that with this book we can share what we have learned over decades of serving youth and families. The first reason for the gratitude comes from having had the opportunity to conduct and publish considerable research that supports the use of family therapy, and to share findings on family processes that are key to the well-being of underserved children and adolescents. We acknowledge the generous funding we received from the National Institutes of Health for development and outcome research. This allowed us to provide free and top-quality treatment to thousands of diverse youth and family members, to learn from families about what works and what does not, and to develop innovations. We have used this knowledge to train the next generation of therapists, researchers, and scholars. We have integrated the voices and perspectives of these thousands of family members into the treatment model we call Culturally Informed and Flexible Family-Based Treatment for Adolescents (CIFFTA). Together we have over 80 years of experience in family processes, family therapy, training, and the role of culture-related processes in adolescent symptoms and treatment. Throughout these years, we have had extraordinary colleagues in centers such as Encuentro, the Spanish Family Guidance Center, and the Center for Family Studies. The pursuit of excellence, passion, and commitment of our colleagues has been inspiring. Although the book is written from the perspective of the clinician, and each chapter is highly practice-oriented, the foundation of our work rests on adolescent, family, and treatment processes that have been supported by rigorous research.

In this book, we make the case for the value of evidence-based treatments (EBTs). It should not be a difficult case to make. If we were considering the use of a powerful medication or undergoing an intensive medical procedure, we would always want to know that the evidence on effectiveness, unintended consequences, and side effects are known and factored into the equation for whether to proceed. No one wants to waste time with ineffective treatments that can make a problem worse, or that leave a patient hopeless because the problem continues a harmful course. The same argument holds for the treatment of mental health problems, such as depression, substance misuse, self-harm, and suicide, especially in children and adolescents. No therapist or parent wants these serious problems to persist and interfere with healthy development. And it would make sense that we do not want to try unproven methods, even if they may be popular. It is a benefit to society that funding agencies are increasingly requiring EBTs for youth and families.

One can argue that the use of treatments proven effective is particularly important in the Latine population (we will say more below about the selection of the term *Latine* instead of *Latino* or *Latinx*), in which many longstanding health disparities have been identified (Alegría et al., 2016). Research has shown that self-harm and suicide risk are high in female/Latina adolescents (Zayas & Gulbas, 2012; Gulbas et al., 2019); that for male/Latine youth, substance use has historically been high in middle school ages (Szapocznik et al., 2007); that severe behavior problems may have particularly harsh legal consequences for Latine youth; that Latine youth and families face difficult conditions due to powerful immigration and acculturation stressors (Cervantes et al., 2014); and that Latine families are less likely to seek and remain in services for their youth (Alegría et al., 2014). It is hard to argue with the premise that Latines and other minoritized populations deserve the best that science has to offer (i.e., EBTs) when treating mental health issues. (In this book, we use *minoritized* to mean a group that is treated as distinct from and less important than the dominant population.) There is no reason why the treatment of depression, self-harm, or substance use should be based on science and evidence any less than the treatment of cancer, hypertension, or diabetes. And yet, the field of Latine youth treatment has been the stage for an intense debate regarding the pros and cons of using EBTs. This is the important *context* in which we present this book, and it is important to acknowledge the best arguments on both sides of this debate.

We must not look upon EBTs with rose-colored glasses. Research methods have limitations, and we should continue to try to improve them and combine different methods (e.g., quantitative and qualitative) to obtain increasingly useful answers. There are two additional well-substantiated problems with EBTs that this book will attempt to address. The first is that manualized treatments have been criticized for being rigid, inflexible, overly restrictive, and prescriptive, and unable to adequately provide guidance in complex clinical situations. The second problem, one even more central to the purpose of this book, is that too many of our current EBTs fail to incorporate what we know about the role of culture and unique life experiences in Latine and other minoritized families. This is the reason for the debate regarding EBTs and the treatment of Latine and other minoritized populations. Treatment manuals in widespread use fail to articulate the precise role of these factors (e.g., worldview and systemic discrimination) *and their impact* on the treatment mechanisms at the core of the manuals. This is particularly problematic given a growing body of evidence on the positive impact of treatments that include culture-related factors within the core of the treatment. These findings suggest that without an integration of cultural factors, even EBTs may not be reaching their optimal outcomes when used with Latine and other diverse clients.

This brings us to a second reason for the gratitude the three of us feel. It comes from being immigrants, or the child of first-generation immigrants, who were welcomed to a generous country that provided us the opportunities to be the first college graduates in our families, leaders in the family therapy field, and the authors of this book. Just as important as our research training and National Institutes of Health–funded research is the fact that our lives were shaped by culture, immigration, and acculturation-related experiences that are described in these pages. We know firsthand that these experiences have powerful impacts on families (i.e., both risk and protective influences), and they helped to shape our sensibilities to these issues. Our parents took great risks, worked harder than anyone should be expected to work, and showed the scars that come from leaving everything behind in their country of birth (often including their parents and other family members whom they never saw again) to begin from scratch in an unfamiliar land.

These experiences helped us to appreciate their role in the process of treatment for Latine and other immigrant groups. When we realized that much of the literature on cultural factors was separate and disconnected from much of the outcome research on adolescent treatment and the manuals for EBTs, we saw the urgent need to share our perspectives on the importance of bridging these two worlds. Too often an EBT that makes no mention of culture when describing its mechanisms expects that the therapist is trained in cultural sensitivity and adds that layer to the treatment in their own idiosyncratic way. We do not believe this is the best approach for the field. We can help therapists be more effective and responsive to the needs of diverse families if the treatment manual itself bridges culture, unique life experiences, and mechanisms. What does this look like concretely? It is a therapist who understands both the power of strong parents who can guide and nurture the youth, and the specific way they may have to do that when the youth is the victim of racism or a traumatic event. The therapist may even have to acknowledge that because the parents continue to experience this same stressor each day, their ability to lead with confidence may be negatively impacted. This is what it looks like to be aware, sensitive, and prepared to tackle therapy mechanisms, culture, and life events simultaneously and in an integrated fashion. When we train and prepare to treat families, we must know as much as possible about family dynamics, family subsystems, and communication so that we are prepared to see clearly and take appropriate steps to help. The same is true of culture, discrimination, immigration, and acculturation—the more we know about how these processes work in a systematic and structural way, and how they negatively impact family relationships, the more prepared we are to help the families we work with.

EVOLVING PERSPECTIVES ON IMMIGRATION

We cannot leave this topic without briefly mentioning the immigration dialogue taking place in many societies. The welcoming of immigrants is never a straight line. Our society goes through peaks and valleys in terms of how receptive it will be to immigrants, and the reception for different groups varies depending on political, social, and economic factors, as well as the history of politics with the country of emigration. Some groups are welcomed with open arms while others are not welcomed at all, even when immigration occurs in the same historical period and for similar reasons. Presently, the mature and informed conversation that should be taking place regarding the most effective processes and rates of planned immigration and naturalization has been replaced by fear, anger, posturing, hostility, and warring factions. It is not something that makes sense, given that the United States continues to need planned immigration to fill positions at all levels of industries and science. This is true because without immigration, the birth rate in the United States continues to decline similar to what is happening in many other countries. In fact, in the most practical terms, we all need more workers contributing taxes on their earnings if we want to have a chance of receiving, when we retire, the benefits we felt we paid for throughout our employment years. There are good points on all sides of the debate, but what is truly needed is a rational and mature conversation.

We share this perspective not to take a political position, but to acknowledge that this is the background, the noise, and the distress that families are experiencing when entering treatment, even as their description of the problem is focused on symptoms such as behavior problems, substance use, or self-harm. As practitioners, we cannot look away from these truths because families that feel they must stay in the shadows will not avail themselves of the services we feel they need to promote well-being. We must also be sensitive to the fact that some individuals who strongly oppose even planned immigration are going through their own difficulties, occupational and culture-related losses, and disillusionment. This distress also goes unacknowledged, though it is quite evident—just look at the increasing suicide rates across race, ethnicity, and economic status profiles. Treatment for individuals and families must also take these painful truths into account. These life experiences are not disconnected from the work of treatment. One cannot treat the presenting problem without understanding the lived experience and the stressors that are impacting symptoms and the family's sense of well-being. We hope that our book shares a perspective on what humane treatment of vulnerable people and their families should look like. We hope it conveys a celebration of all diversity so that the beauty and strength of differences can be better appreciated and mobilized in treatment. We also hope what we share will help you *see* your client more clearly. It is certainly a wise adage that "If we see clearly, we will know what to do."

TERMINOLOGY

In this final section, we would like to share our thoughts on terminology and labels that we use throughout the book. We begin with a brief overview of the individuals included under the Hispanic and Latine umbrella, including the terminology of *Hispanic*, *Latino*, and *Latinx*. One of the most popular umbrella terms to be used widely in the United States was *Hispanic*. Hispanic came into widespread use in the 1970s and was included in the 1980 census. The term was welcomed in large part because it brought together a large group of individuals claiming roots in Spanish-speaking countries. The considerable size of the group under this umbrella had important implications for the group's political power and led to an appreciation of the group's growing influence in American culture.

In the decade of the 1990s, a sense arose that *Hispanic* overemphasized links to Spain (and the problematic parts of Spain's history of conquest) and descendants from Spanish-speaking countries. Use of the term *Latino* gained more widespread appeal. *Latino* was considered to accentuate important roots in the countries of Latin America. Its emphasis was on the history and experiences of people who had been in Latin America long before the arrival of Spaniards. For the past decades, the terms *Latino* and *Hispanic* have tended to be used interchangeably, and they appeared together for the first time in the 2000 census. The fact that the terms are often used interchangeably does not mean that there are not strong emotional arguments for the use of one over another.

One of the more recent terms to hit the scene is *Latinx*. It has been recommended as a more inclusive term that refers to individuals of Latin American descent without placing emphasis on issues of gender (especially male gender, as in *Latino*) and excluding individuals who prefer not to be identified by traditional gender status. This gender-neutral term has not yet caught on among the population it is meant to represent. Only 25% of individuals of Latine descent are familiar with the *Latinx* term, and only 3% use *Latinx* to describe themselves (Noe-Bustamante et al., 2020). Perhaps the reluctance to accept the terms should not be surprising given that the population tends to be more on the conservative and traditional side of the continuum, and that Spanish is a "gendered" language. For example, the words *el libro* and *el capítulo*, meaning the book and the chapter, respectively, are linked to male gender, while *palabras*, meaning the words, are linked to female gender. This may contribute to a reluctance to see the need for a gender-neutral term. Perhaps it is just too soon in the life of the new terminology. Indeed, according to a Pew 2020 survey (Noe-Bustamante et al., 2020), even the term *Latino* is not as commonly endorsed as the original *Hispanic*. This brings us to the term *Latine,* which we have chosen for this book. It is akin to the gender-neutral term for a student, which is *estudiante*. As we were reaching a decision on whether to use Hispanic, Latino, or Latinx, we found a compelling set of arguments for the use of *Latine*. This term is being widely used in Spanish-language literature and is more in tune with a gender-neutral term a Spanish-speaking person might use. We chose to use this term, but we also acknowledge that we are unsure about whether it will stand the test of time.

In general, Mexicans, Puerto Ricans, Cubans, Spaniards, and Nicaraguans will typically want to be called by their identity as relates to the name of their home country. They identify most with their country of origin and not really with any of the umbrella terms. Of course, some may prefer Mexican American or Cuban American. Many would not be happy with a hyphenated label such as Mexican-American, which can convey that they are not fully American. Individuals acknowledge the similarities they share, but they also appreciate the substantial differences in the reasons for and route of historical and current migration, reception in the United States, traditionalism, social class, education, and other life experiences (marginalization and immigration-related separations). The experience of a Mexican American whose family has been in New Mexico for three generations, or a Puerto Rican whose family has been living on the island for the same amount of time, may differ across myriad dimensions from that of a Venezuelan or a Honduran who has been in the United States for 4 months. While it is common to use such general categories as *Hispanic* or *Latino* or *Latine,* for the sake of convenience and to attempt to point to commonalities shared by a larger group of people, it is important to keep in mind the substantial limitations of any such categorical label.

REASONS AND ROUTES OF MIGRATION TO THE UNITED STATES

As we describe in more detail in Chapter 2, there are myriad reasons for migration. Of course, any such discussion must begin with a subset of Latines of Mexican descent, for whom the question is not "How did they come to the United States?" but "How did the United States come to them?" Before the early 19th century, most of the people of Mexico were of mixed Spanish and Indigenous background. After approximately 300 years of Spanish rule, Mexico won its independence in 1821. For the inhabitants of Northern Mexico, however, everything changed when war erupted between Mexico and the United States in 1846. When Mexico lost the war, they also lost land that is now Texas, California, and other sections of the Southwest. With that, and with a later land sale by Mexico to the United States, one-third of Mexico became the United States and *close to 100,000 Mexicans were suddenly living in the United States without ever leaving their homes.* These Mexican families were now susceptible to being called foreigners by anyone who did not understand history, territorial expansion, land conquest, and land sales. This history and its consequences continue to be the roots of present-day tensions.

TYPE OF IMMIGRANTS

John Berry (2006), one of the foremost writers on migration and acculturation, describes different types of migrants including voluntary immigrants, refugees, asylum seekers, and sojourners. It is beneficial to think about the difference between individuals in these categories, but the overlap is considerable, and people placed in one category may argue that they belong elsewhere.

Voluntary immigrants are those individuals who migrate away from their country of origin by choice. They are said to be in search of improved educational, economic, and employment opportunities. There is a great deal of variability in terms of how these immigrants are received and welcomed in the United States.

Refugees do not leave their countries voluntarily or by choice but are displaced by violence and persecution. Refugees are often welcomed into the host country, and their entry is documented in agreements that invite the refugees to stay. Refugees are often characterized by a desire to return to their country of origin when it becomes safe to do so.

Many people who are said to have come *voluntarily* will point out the great turmoil, danger, and persecution that they were fleeing. Whether or not government agreements were in place does not change the danger that the family experienced and that led them to leave everything they owned, everyone they loved, the land, the town squares where families cared for each other, and the community that gave their lives meaning.

Asylum seekers also request refuge in a new country due to fear of persecution and violence. Again, you see that the boundaries between these categories of immigrants are quite vague and susceptible to interpretation. And yet, they are important because the categorization leads some groups to feel they have more of a right to be in the United States than others, and they may become unsupportive of immigrants who they feel do not have a "good enough" reason to want to enter the United States.

Those immigrants who are made to feel unwelcome may forever feel separate and may be less likely to incorporate themselves into society. There may be an important difference between immigrants who do not see a return to their homeland in their future, that is, those who are said to "burn their bridges behind them," and those who either return regularly or never fully disconnect from their families back home. The latter group can often be described as transnational, with their identities connected to more than one nation.

To know a Latine family fully, one must be able to distinguish these different lived experiences and be open to the stories that a family shares about themselves, the life-changing decisions they have made for their families, and their place in the world. These subtle differences in life experiences are often connected to strong emotions and pain or pride in the client. This book is written for those who are willing to truly prepare themselves to be as effective as possible with their clients no matter what background they come from. Although the research began with Latine clients and the need to integrate culture and science, it is now about a template for integrating the lived experience of many diverse clients and the science on family and treatment process.

OUR USE OF PRONOUNS

We should also mention our approach to the use of pronouns and our attempts to ensure that our writing is as gender inclusive as possible. Guidelines on language (e.g., American Psychological Association, the *Chicago Manual of Style*, and the Modern Language Association) support the movement away from gender-restrictive terms such as *he* and *she* and toward the use of the singular *they*. Whenever we must use a pronoun and the correct one is unknown, we use the singular *they*. Some will argue that this usage is not grammatically correct but as the rules on grammar have evolved, experts have argued that this usage is grammatically correct. This of course does not guarantee that our grandchild will not one day pick up the book and still say, "What were they thinking?", because new and more useful and inclusive guidelines have evolved.

ROADMAP FOR THE BOOK

This book can be broken down into three main parts. In the first part, consisting of Chapters 1 through 3, we summarize the diverse literature that has created a foundation for our work. In the second part, Chapters 4 through 8, we provide a deep dive into each of the CIFFTA treatment components, details on the *nuts and bolts* of delivery, and a clearer sense of the available tools that CIFFTA offers. We also present a chapter including case studies that bring clinical situations and interventions to life. In the third part of the book, consisting of Chapters 9 and 10, we document the strategies we have used to expand our work beyond Latine families to include other diverse populations. We also document the strategies we have used to address the challenges the field faces regarding family intervention training, adoption, implementation, and sustainability.

This book is not a treatment manual and does not provide all the requisite training and materials needed to generate optimal outcomes and high fidelity when implementing CIFFTA. The book does provide a strong foundation for family-based work with Latine adolescents, a general description of the CIFFTA components, and guidelines for implementation. Access to the full array of CIFFTA tools, including the treatment manual and psychoeducational modules, is available as part of a training contract with Training and Implementation Associates. (Follow this link for details about our training program: *www.guilford.com/santisteban-materials*.) Trainees receive online access to a treatment manual, dozens of downloadable psychoeducational modules in PDF form on different treatment topics and in English and Spanish, animations that help demonstrate effective intervention delivery, and implementation and fidelity tools. Training can typically be completed in 12–15 hours, and a 6-month period of expert consultation and coaching is highly recommended as therapists begin CIFFTA implementation.

Contents

I. FOUNDATIONS OF LATINE YOUTH AND FAMILY TREATMENT

1. The Treatment of Latine Youth and Families — 3
2. The Latine Experience: Unique Stressors, Resilience, and Tools for Systematic Assessment — 20
   with Richard C. Cervantes
3. Foundations of Effective Treatment of Latine Youth and Families — 38

II. CIFFTA PRACTICE GUIDE

4. Preparing the Ground for CIFFTA Implementation — 59
5. CIFFTA Individual Therapy with the Adolescent — 86
6. CIFFTA Therapy with the Entire Family — 106
7. CIFFTA's Psychoeducational and Modular Component — 135
8. Case Examples Showing CIFFTA in Action — 159

III. BROADER CLINICAL CONSIDERATIONS

9. Training, Implementation, and Sustainability 191
with Alejandra C. Santisteban

10. Extensions to New Populations, Unique Applications, and Future Directions for CIFFTA 209

References 223

Index 239

FOUNDATIONS OF LATINE YOUTH AND FAMILY TREATMENT

1

The Treatment of Latine Youth and Families

Behavioral treatments make a significant difference in the lives of children and adolescents by reducing disruptive behaviors, depression, anxiety, substance misuse, self-harm, and suicide-related behavior. These approaches can reduce presenting symptoms, increase child and adolescent well-being, and minimize disruptions to their healthy development. Ameliorating emotional and behavioral problems during an already complex child and adolescent stage of development can have a long-lasting impact on a youth's well-being.

Many successful treatments that ameliorate presenting symptoms have also focused on identifying and modifying the underlying factors that contribute to the emergence and maintenance of the symptoms. Family-based interventions focus on reducing underlying family risk factors while enhancing protective factors. Family therapy has been found to be particularly efficacious for treating a variety of disorders including attention-deficit/hyperactivity disorder (ADHD), depression, disruptive behaviors, and substance use (Kaslow et al., 2012; Hogue et al., 2021; Van Ryzin et al., 2016; Vermeulen-Smit et al., 2015; Mena et al., 2023; Santisteban et al., 2011, 2017, 2022; Sheidow et al., 2022). Family interventions can have an effect long after the therapist is gone by transforming maladaptive family-level conditions (e.g., family conflict, ruptured relationships) and mobilizing protective family factors and relationships (e.g., support, validation, and nurturance). Once an entire family is strengthened and made healthier, even other siblings/youth and family members not currently in treatment can reap the benefits of a better-functioning family. Furthermore, when a therapist succeeds at engaging family members as allies in treatment, the work becomes easier. It strengthens the caregiver's leadership role, and they work collaboratively to effect change for the family system both in sessions and at home.

A great strength of family therapy models is that they take a contextual or relational approach. This means that the therapist attempts to understand an individual's behavior, at least in part, as a result of the relationship dynamics that surround it. The relationships can elicit or constrain certain behaviors (e.g., family members can restrict the discussion of past traumatic experiences), and the behavior can send an important relational message (e.g., cry for help or a refusal to accept constraints). The therapist will use the relationship context to better understand and even modify individual behaviors. Throughout this book, the relational approach also guides us in reflecting on the complex contexts (i.e., schools, neighborhoods, and health systems) that directly impact the behaviors of both adolescents and families.

When working with Latine and other diverse families, we also appreciate the value of *culturally centered* treatments. Such approaches put culture-related material at the core of the treatment and have been associated with superior outcomes (Hall et al., 2016; Soto et al., 2018) when used with diverse populations. Such treatments integrate assumptions, metaphors, and worldviews that are consistent with those endorsed by the diverse clients and may be better able to address such factors as trauma, discrimination, immigration and acculturation stress, and other culture-related stressors (Bernal & Domenech Rodriguez, 2012; Cervantes et al., 2018). The contextual perspective used in family therapy facilitates the identification of systemic and structural inequities that work against youth and family well-being. Approaching the presenting problem from this perspective also provides thoughtful ways of helping the family to address these stressors. The ability to incorporate cultural values and worldviews into the therapy process has been a hallmark of family therapy (Boyd-Franklin, 2010; Falicov, 2014; McGoldrick & Hardy, 2019) though we have argued that this strength has not always filtered into the more formal evidence-based treatments (EBTs; Santisteban et al., 2013). Treatments that integrate cultural domains may better address the unique life experiences that contribute to hopelessness, stressors, symptom emergence and maintenance, and poor service utilization, retention, and treatment outcomes (Abraído-Lanza et al., 2016). These experiences should be a starting point in the conceptualization of both symptom emergence and return to more adaptive functioning. Treatments designed to identify and work through the powerful everyday stressors experienced by Latine and other minoritized clients will be perceived as more relevant and helpful by the client. Working from this perspective means that culture-related experiences and mechanisms of change are two threads running through the same discussion and therapeutic work.

This position is vastly different from those who argue that it is best to focus primarily on the mechanisms of action of the therapy and to separately add a layer of cultural competence or cultural sensitivity in the delivery of the services. The latter argument assumes that culture-related factors are peripheral to the principal targets of treatment and change. We argue, in contrast, that culture is always present in therapy, but it is often unacknowledged. The worldview of the dominant culture is already (quietly and subtly) the foundation of the generic treatments and arguments for "culture-free" treatment mechanisms. The cultural assumptions behind the generic treatments are a perfect fit for the dominant group. From that perspective, *cultural competence* is easily seen as an added layer that must later be placed atop an established clinical approach, to address the treatment of the patient or family from a minority or nonmainstream culture. Traditionally, in manuals that delineate generic clinical approaches, there is little mention of how the main components and mechanisms central to how the treatment works (e.g., cognitions, interpersonal relationships, definition of family, communication, hierarchy, ecological/contextual processes) are directly impacted by diverse cultural factors. The only way to explain how cultural nuances can be left out of the core explanation of these treatments is that nuances of the dominant, mainstream culture were *assumed,* as a foundation of the treatments' driving theory and associated practices, but never acknowledged as such.

An example of these subtle assumptions became evident when Latine families were found to fall short in their mission to support the autonomy and individuality of a child and were prematurely labeled *enmeshed* or *overinvolved*. A Latine would consider it impossible to talk about family mechanisms of action without talking about what *familia* means. These parents did not get the memo on the urgency of successful *launching* by a certain age, often around 18 years. It was taken as a given that families should prioritize the separation and autonomy of teens as they move toward young adulthood. That was an assumption of the dominant culture so widely accepted as to not require discussion. This prioritization of autonomy sometimes led therapists to emphasize the need for individual therapy that excluded family members who were not allowing timely separation and individuation. Yet we often heard Latine families who endorsed the priority of family involvement and other aspects of familism complain that the therapy approach was misguided. A similar conflict can arise when therapists encourage adolescents to speak their minds in therapy, and express whatever things they dislike about their families. In traditional Latine and even Haitian families in which hierarchy is important, parents may feel a therapist who encourages such behavior (which they view as disrespectful) is misguided. Suggesting that the teen speak freely goes against the expectation of *respeto* (respect) in the family.

Interestingly, because values, beliefs, and cultural norms are not static, we might be able to detect changes in mainstream thinking that are likely to influence what we as therapists convey is a new normal. For example, now that more *mainstream* families are struggling with inflation, housing shortages, and high student loans, more individuals are living with their parents well into their 20s and even 30s. This may be contributing to a change in mainstream dialogue, which now includes the term *emerging adults*. This term helps to normalize what might once have been labeled a failure to launch.

To provide a balanced view, we should also look at the other side of the divide—scholars and clinicians who highlight the rich and diverse experiences and culture-bound aspects of Latine clients but may prematurely disregard EBTs. Many in this camp can correctly point out the substantial limitations of EBTs that fail to account for culture. However, when taken to an extreme, the ill-advised response is to pay lip service to the value of available EBTs while promoting less proven treatments that highlight only the role of culture. These may be treatments that are culturally sensitive but totally lacking in evidence of their efficacy, effectiveness, or impact on established mechanisms of change. Discarding the benefits of EBTs because they fail to incorporate cultural considerations is the proverbial "throwing out the baby with the bath water." Alternative non-EBTs may provide a good fit with the expectations and preferences of Latine clients, but they have not done the work of integrating accepted knowledge on the best-established change mechanisms and therapeutic processes. We argue that a therapy that fits with the client's cultural worldview is *necessary but not sufficient*. Optimally, we should integrate advances in treatment, findings from process research, and insights from ethnic psychology (Foxen, 2016)—and avoid the vilification or disregard for one side or the other.

CULTURALLY INFORMED AND FLEXIBLE FAMILY-BASED TREATMENT FOR ADOLESCENTS

The treatment set forth in this book, Culturally Informed and Flexible Family-Based Treatment for Adolescents (CIFFTA), is designed to achieve a high level of integration of knowledge pertaining to adolescent, family, and cultural processes. It is an EBT that depends on well-established therapy mechanisms (e.g., family systems, motivation enhancement, adolescent skills) while also integrating cultural complexity and nuance at its core. We make the case that to focus on the more generic "melting-pot" concoction is to disregard some of the most powerful risk factors at work on adolescents and families. Also disregarded are powerful protective factors that a therapist can use to help Latine families. We contend that treatment manuals that disregard culture and lived experience are not the most effective tools, because they ignore the unique circumstances and events that are most real in the daily lives of many minoritized groups. It also reminds us that there is no "one-size-fits-all" Latine either. The therapist must be attuned to the uniqueness of the experiences of each individual and family.

CIFFTA was developed with the goal of taking the best that EBTs and Latine psychology have to offer and creating a comprehensive family-based approach for Latine youth and families. CIFFTA recognizes and incorporates the advances and innovations achieved by dedicated researchers and theorists on both sides of the aforementioned debate. And in fact, CIFFTA has been criticized for being too "research-based" as well as being too "focused on Latine cultural factors"—an indicator that it may be lodged in exactly the right space. At its best, research serves to amplify the voices of the diverse populations we serve and to ensure that their life experiences and worldviews are integrated into systems that are designed to serve them in the most effective way possible. If the reader can analyze CIFFTA and discern both the generic mechanisms that are well established in family systems theory *and* the way that the life experiences of Latine youth and families are intertwined with theoretical individual and family mechanisms, then this book will have served its purpose.

CIFFTA encompasses three major innovations: (1) creating a multicomponent treatment and creating synergy between its family treatment, child/adolescent treatment, and psychoeducational components; (2) making cultural themes central to the treatment manual, training, and coaching while linking them to core therapy mechanisms; and (3) creating a flexible and adaptive modular framework that allows the treatment to be tailored to the unique clinical and cultural characteristics of youth and families. In the next section, we explain each in a bit more detail.

The Family Component

CIFFTA has *family work* at its core because the family is one of the most powerful contexts in which child and adolescent development takes place. Risk factors, protective factors, guidance, socialization, and the nurturance of healthy child and adolescent development occur in families. Family processes can mobilize, constrain, shine a light on, or conceal individual strengths and weaknesses. There is an impressive amount of research on family processes, and research has supported the efficacy of family therapy when addressing adolescent symptoms such as conduct and behavior problems and substance use. The family is the context in which a vast number of life's most intense behavior-shaping experiences occur, and even as autonomy and differentiation processes can become prominent in a youth's life, the family continues to be highly influential. CIFFTA answers the question "Who is family?" with a flexible definition of family that includes traditional, extended, and elected families. CIFFTA includes the entire network of support and resources that can be utilized during treatment. We are free to mobilize the pastor, the coach, the godmother, the neighbor, and the school counselor who can stand by and support healthy change. Chapter 6 will provide further information on the "nuts and bolts" of family intervention delivery. CIFFTA zooms in on specific techniques and strategies for mobilizing family support, validation, and protection while reducing negativity, disengagement/neglect, and other risk factors.

The Individual Therapy Component

CIFFTA reflects a substantial departure from the senior authors' previous work on a different family treatment model (Brief Strategic Family Therapy), which was restricted to conjoint family therapy and typically delivered in a once-per-week format (Santisteban et al., 2003, 2006). Although family intervention is indeed a powerful foundation for the treatment of adolescents, we believe adolescents also benefit from an individually oriented treatment component that can help them with the complex tasks that emerge during the adolescent stage of development. Developmentally appropriate interventions include motivation enhancement, goal setting, working through sexual orientation and gender identity questions, and teaching interpersonal effectiveness and emotion regulation skills. In our work with adolescents who turned to substance misuse to cope with emotional turmoil and life stressors (Santisteban et al., 2011) or turned to self-harm due to the marginalization that comes from coming out as an LGBTQ+ youth (Mena et al., 2024a), it became clear that there is a need to contribute to healthy adolescent development using one-on-one sessions with the youth. This is particularly true with older adolescents who are struggling to develop effective skills for leading their own lives in a healthy direction. It is overly limiting to reach the adolescent only through the family and not directly. As we show later in this book, this does not preclude the issues that emerge in individual therapy from being processed within the family, when the timing is optimal.

For these reasons, our effort to improve the outcomes of our family-based treatment included the integration of *individual* work into CIFFTA in a way that complements and enhances the family work. For example, most youngsters with substance abuse problems are accustomed to being strongly confronted by adults in the family, school, legal, and treatment systems in a disempowering way. It became particularly important to consider EBTs designed to help adolescents develop their own goals and motivation for change without triggering the defensive and *stonewalling* stance that confrontation tends to elicit. The growing evidence that Motivational Interviewing (MI) strategies could be extraordinarily successful in lowering adolescent resistance (Miller & Rollnick, 2023) and that MI could be successfully combined with other treatments led to its integration into our work. CIFFTA interventions also sought to strengthen the often weak set of life skills adolescents bring into treatment. Interpersonal effectiveness and emotion regulation skills (Linehan, 2014a, 2014b, in press-a, in press-b; Santisteban et al., 2015) are critically important when working with struggling youth. Individual sessions can facilitate the generalization of psychoeducational material, teaching them emotion modulation or interpersonal effectiveness skills that can make a difference in the youth's daily challenges in multiple settings (e.g., peers, family). Finally, the individually focused treatment sessions allowed an exploration of the youth's identity on issues such as ethnicity, race, sexual orientation, and gender identity. It is common for second-generation immigrant teens (those born in the United States) to have perspectives on the traditions of their country and culture of origin that are quite different from those of their first-generation parents and grandparents. The same can be true with feelings and attitudes about gender identity and sexual orientation, which may not be accepted by their parents and grandparents and the larger Latine culture.

Sometimes an adolescent must explore parts of themselves before they are ready to explain them to family members. These topics may be avoided in the early stages of family therapy because of the intensity of the conflicts and the hurtful attacks that may result. Some therapists see these attacks and decide they must exclude the family completely. That is a mistake. Individual sessions with teens allow them a chance to discuss and explore all these issues, and the therapist can then plan with the teen on how best to process these issues effectively in family sessions. Individual sessions with teens can also include a full discussion of strategies for handling the stress resulting from the discrimination and alienation they experience. In short, our assumption is that therapists can work to improve the family context in which adolescents find themselves, while also working directly with youngsters struggling with the challenging demands of the adolescent developmental stage. Chapter

5 provides a more detailed discussion of the delivery of individual treatment in CIFFTA.

The Psychoeducational Component

The third CIFFTA component consists of structured psychoeducational modules delivered in a didactic format. A major assumption behind the development of this component is that there is a great deal of material on such issues as substance use, self-harm, social media, discrimination, acculturation processes, parenting practices, family acceptance following LGBTQ+ disclosure, and legal system involvement that may be highly relevant to certain families, but that is also complex and difficult to digest. Psychoeducational sessions are helpful because the free-flowing process of therapy does not always allow time to focus on the family's learning and integration of these important facts. Psychoeducational sessions provide a structured and systematic presentation of important topics in a format and at a level that parents and the adolescent could more readily absorb. This information serves to normalize the issues because it shows that they emerge in many families. Families can sit back and hear the information and decide whether it relates to them and how. Furthermore, the modular structure of this material facilitates the specific family *tailoring* approach that is important to CIFFTA. Only those modules that address an important content area for a given family are selected and integrated into their treatment plan. Based on individual sessions with the teen, certain modules may be selected as relevant (for instance, trauma or self-harm). Using the modules is a less emotionally evocative and personal way to introduce issues that are of high relevance to the youth. Youth and families can also participate in the selection of the module using a shared decision-making approach. Chapter 7 provides more information on the module's details and delivery process.

Creation of Synergy between Treatment Components

Each of CIFFTA's components can stand alone, but the full effect of the treatment is achieved only when you actively and intentionally create synergy and bridges among them. An example of bridging the components is the *generalization* work that follows any didactic psychoeducational module. Generalization helps clients with the difficult task of integrating new knowledge and skills into their daily lives. For example, in CIFFTA's psychoeducational work, a family may learn about the multifaceted and predictable impact that acculturation or immigration-related separations can have on family relationships. The processes are normalized, discussed as they happen across many families, and can be absorbed with less defensiveness. In therapy sessions, the family returns to this topic and processes how these dynamics play out in their own home and how they can use what was learned to relate to each other differently. A family that learns in psychoeducational sessions that it is normal for a child who has been separated from parents to experience sadness, resentment, a sense of loss and abandonment, and to have a need to ask difficult questions, gets to explore and validate all these feelings with their own child in a family session. The therapist helps shape the family interactions to facilitate the healthy processing of the issue. An adolescent who learns interpersonal effectiveness skills in a psychoeducational session can be coached on how to use them effectively with peers in individual therapy sessions and can be coached *in vivo* on how to use the skills with the parents and siblings in family therapy sessions. A family therapy session can be the arena in which parents can be taught to support (rather than dismiss or challenge) new and emerging adolescent behaviors and new skills learned via psychoeducation (e.g., communication, emotion regulation). Conversely, a family session in which an adolescent blows up and hurts their own cause can be a learning opportunity and can lead to an extension of a skills session that focuses on why the skill (e.g., interpersonal effectiveness skills) did not work within that family session and how to handle the incident more effectively in the future. This is what we call bridging the work between the complementary treatment components to achieve CIFFTA's optimal effect.

Integration of Cultural Themes into CIFFTA's Therapy Mechanisms

CIFFTA sets culture-related content and issues alongside established treatment mechanisms. We seek to avoid the mistakes of the past that allowed two bodies of information (on culture and on family therapy mechanisms) to exist in separate silos that a competent therapist must struggle to bridge in their own idiosyncratic way. Keeping these two bodies of knowledge separate and apart deprives the therapist of some of the richest and most useful tools available (Santisteban et al., 2013). The richness of family system concepts is most evident when considering the variety of experiences and relationships encountered by individuals of diverse backgrounds. Likewise, the complex relationships and contextual interactions that occur in minoritized individuals' lives can be better appreciated by looking at them through the lens of systemic principles and mechanisms.

When treating a Latine family with its unique and powerful life experiences, values, beliefs, behaviors, and help-seeking patterns, one of the first questions that emerge is about the fit between the assumptions, tools, content, and processes that define that model and those that define the culture of the client and family. The challenge is to articulate the relevance and precise links between culture-related factors and established family concepts and processes. The CIFFTA therapist is trained to ask questions such as:

- How does acculturation impact parenting practices and communication?
- How does an immigration-related parent–child separation impact the relationship quality in the recently reunited family?
- How do the norms regarding *respeto* (respect) and adherence to hierarchy in a traditional family dictate how disagreements can be handled at home and in a therapy session?
- How might a therapist who encourages an adolescent to confront his traditional and hierarchical father be violating the expectations and norms of the father and family?
- How does an expectation that a couple *must* have an egalitarian relationship violate the norms of some very traditional and non-egalitarian couples? How do we strengthen each member's voice in this context?
- How can a healthy family, strong parenting practices, and socialization help to buffer youth from racist experiences in the world?

These types of questions link culture and diverse worldviews to established family processes and mechanisms. They are how we determine which cultural factors to highlight when seeking key changes. Falicov (2014) reminds us that in considering cultural differences, it is critically important to identify *those differences that make a difference*. That is, the therapist will be able to identify many culture-related issues but must focus on those differences between people that are particularly relevant to understanding differences in treatment relevance, processes, and outcomes.

For example, Latine families are said to highly endorse *familism* or the obligation to protect, support, and always consider the family (Sabogal et al., 1987). A family that highly endorses familism may be less likely to connect with a treatment that is highly individually oriented, that excludes family members, and that does not interpret behaviors in relation to their impact on the family. The advice of a provider that the client *do what is right for them as an individual, without worrying about the family's reaction*, may not hit fertile ground without more processing of how family obligation and guarding the family name is a deeply ingrained value in that client. The work of healthy differentiation must take the client's ingrained perspective on familism into account.

And no, the individual's continued orientation to the family is not necessarily a sign of immaturity and lack of individuation.

Our previous research on culture and family processes led to interesting findings that impact the therapy process. These include:

- How the level of acculturation of parents can impact the way they conduct their parenting and the efficacy of those parenting practices in helping youth to stay away from behavior problems (Santisteban et al., 2012). We found that parents who endorsed more of the *Hispanic culture from their country of origin* reported more involvement as part of their parenting practices and lower behavior problems in their youth.

- How Latine parents reported discomfort with the concepts, terminology, and lack of information concerning sexual behavior and safe sex, and that this was in large part associated with their discomfort in having these conversations with their kids (Mena et al., 2008a). This is particularly important given that prevention specialists have shown that having this conversation is one way parents can be helpful in reducing risk in youth.

- How immigration-related parent–child separations can be associated with relationship difficulties during reunification (Mena et al., 2008b), how this process can lead to depressive symptoms in youth, especially Latina youth (Mena et al., 2023), and how it can be addressed in treatment (Santisteban et al., 2013).

- How Latine culture and religiosity, both of which are considered powerful protective factors, can make it even more difficult for many Latine parents to validate and accept their LGBTQ+ youth (Mena et al., 2024a).

These are all examples of how treatment can make itself truly relevant to the reality of the Latine family by ensuring that the therapist has specialized content ready to address these types of situations.

An Adaptive and Flexible Framework

Youth and families enter treatment with different strengths and areas for growth, varied presenting problems and co-occurring disorders, myriad family constellations and structures, and diverse culture-related characteristics and experiences. Given this reality, there is no one-size-fits-all approach to treatment, no matter how comprehensive the treatment manual is. There should be no question that the process of adaptation and tailoring the generic techniques to the specific family will take place in one form or another. The question is whether the adaptations and tailoring will occur out in the open in a way that is replicable, or behind closed doors in a way that is very idiosyncratic. CIFFTA's approach is to spell out within the manual as much of the adaptation and tailoring process as possible. *It seeks to place as much attention on the tailoring process as it does on the main therapy mechanisms.*

Any treatment can claim to be flexible by allowing individual therapists to make adaptations or enhancements in idiosyncratic ways. The problem is that such adaptations can later be criticized for undermining the fidelity needed to achieve an optimal outcome. Any unplanned and nonsystematic changes made by a therapist make it difficult to know what was really delivered to a client, and these hidden modifications make the complete treatment package difficult to replicate. The benefit that comes with an adaptive treatment is flexibility guided by decision rules that can be clearly articulated in the manual and, if followed, can simultaneously create flexibility and facilitate replication. CIFFTA's adaptive approach resembles what Sue (2006) called *dynamic sizing*. The important caveat is that CIFFTA seeks to provide decision rules for the sizing and tailoring so that it can be done in a systematic and replicable fashion.

CIFFTA's use of an adaptive framework is facilitated by our group of approximately 20 (to date) psychoeducational modules that can be delivered to youth and parents in English or Spanish, and that include information on prominent issues that have emerged in our 30 years of working with Latine youth and families. Flexible treatments with well-defined options seek to include in a manualized treatment the wisdom of the highly qualified and culturally competent clinician.

One important result of the flexible framework is that it facilitates a *transdiagnostic* approach. It helps CIFFTA avoid the pitfalls related to being an approach that focuses on only one symptom and facilitates the process of addressing many different symptoms within a broader category of problems roughly described as a "youth behavior problem syndrome" (Jessor & Jessor, 1977). Transdiagnostic treatments seek to address "maintaining mechanisms" that may underlie several, often co-occurring disorders (McHugh et al., 2009). In CIFFTA these maintaining mechanisms include family maladaptive relationship patterns, invalidation, high conflict, and emotion dysregulation. A transdiagnostic approach allows for flexibility to make systematic adjustments for prespecified conditions (Kendall et al., 2008) and begins to address the concern that manualized EBTs are overly rigid manuals and narrow in their focus. EBTs that can only be shown to work with one narrow type of diagnosis or presenting problem are unlikely to be attractive or sustainable in the front lines of practice given that comorbidity and co-occurring disorders are the rule and not the exception.

Evidence of CIFFTA's Efficacy and Effectiveness

A program of research funded by a series of National Institute of Health grants led to the development and rigorous testing of CIFFTA for minoritized adolescents and families. We are indebted to the National Institute on Drug Abuse (NIDA), the National Institute on Minority Health and Health Disparities (NIMHD), and the National Institute on Mental Health (NIMH) for their leadership and funding to help effective treatments reach our communities. An early NIDA study (Santisteban et al., 2011) helped to develop the CIFFTA components and provide a preliminary test of its efficacy. The study used an "add-on" design to isolate the effects attributable to the enhancements, so it compared participants assigned to a family therapy-only condition and a family therapy plus CIFFTA components. The study included Latine adolescents who met criteria for substance abuse disorder as outlined in the fourth edition, text revision of the *Diagnostic and Statistical Manual of Mental Disorders* (DSM-IV-TR; American Psychiatric Association [APA], 2000). Most youth had substantial marijuana and alcohol use and to a lesser extent cocaine use when they entered treatment. Change was investigated between baseline and an 8-month follow-up assessment.

Santisteban et al. (2011) Study Details

Twenty-four adolescents and their families were randomly assigned to either the experimental treatment (CIFFTA) or traditional family therapy (TFT). Below are findings from the study.

- Adolescents in CIFFTA showed a significantly greater reduction in self-reported drug use (marijuana + cocaine), $F(1, 22) = 10.59, p < .01, \eta^2 = .33$, compared to the TFT condition.
- Self-reported change in drug use was consistent with urine analysis results.
- Adolescents in CIFFTA reported a significantly greater improvement in parenting practices, $F(1, 22) = 9.01, p < .01, \eta^2 = .29$.

These results showed the promise of an adaptive and culturally informed treatment for substance misuse in Latine adolescents.

A second study funded by NIMHD (Santisteban et al., 2017) was designed to test a computer-assisted version of the CIFFTA model. As part of an ongoing program of treatment improvement, our team investigated the possible benefits of integrating technology-assisted intervention into the existing CIFFTA approach. Technology-assisted treatments can enhance the attractiveness of an intervention, particularly for youth, and can aid in the intervention process by (1) requiring fewer hours of counselor contact (which lowers cost and stress on agency system resources); (2) increasing the client's therapeutic work between sessions; (3) reducing the logistical barriers (e.g., travel time, public transportation) that often plague low-income clients; (4) offering key treatment components delivered via videos in a standardized manner to maintain fidelity; and (5) providing variable information formats (e.g., multimedia) that make the intervention more engaging. These features appeared particularly promising in the context of CIFFTA because technology could support an adaptive and modular framework (e.g., facilitating the selection of only modules that are relevant to the unique needs of an identified adolescent and family).

Santisteban et al. (2017) Study Details

Eighty Latine and African American youth and families were randomized to either immediate computer-assisted CIFFTA or delayed computer-assisted CIFFTA. The findings below represent significant between-groups effects showing the superiority of the immediate computer-assisted CIFFTA condition when compared to the delayed condition that received no treatment during the same period. Compared to families in the delayed condition, families receiving treatment immediately showed superior outcomes. More specifically, for immediate CIFFTA:

- Parents reported significant reductions in youth conduct disorder ($B = -5.17$, $SE = 1.73$, $p < .01$, confidence interval $= [-8.55, -1.79]$).
- Parents reported significant reductions in youth socialized aggression (or peer-based delinquency) ($B = -2.04$, $SE = 0.83$, $p < .05$, confidence interval $= [-3.67, -0.41]$).
- Parents report significant improvements in family cohesion ($B = 1.34$, $SE = 0.50$, $p < .01$, confidence interval $= [.36, 2.32]$).
- Youth reported significant reductions in externalizing problems ($B = -4.22$, $SE = 1.40$, $p < .01$, confidence interval $= [-6.95, -1.48]$).
- Youth reported significant improvements in family cohesion ($B = 1.31$, $SE = 0.46$, $p < .01$, confidence interval $= [0.41, 2.21]$).

Baseline to 6-week posttreatment (T1–T3) analyses showed that these significant within-subject effects were sustained for the treatment group. When the delayed-condition families received the computer-assisted CIFFTA, they also showed improved outcomes. Results highlight that adolescent behavior problems can be significantly impacted by a computer-assisted intervention that replaces some face-to-face meetings with computer-delivered psychoeducational modules.

A third and larger trial funded by the NIMHD (Santisteban et al., 2022) tested CIFFTA with youth reporting behavior problems and sought to expand knowledge on culturally sensitive treatments with a randomized controlled trial. Specifically, we investigated CIFFTA's ability to engage and retain Latine youth and families, to modify family functioning, and to reduce adolescent internalizing and externalizing symptoms. The study also sought to investigate the role that acculturation may play in treatment outcomes. Assessment occurred at baseline prior to treatment and then again after 16 weeks of intervention.

Santisteban et al. (2022) Study Details

The study in which 200 Latine adolescents 11–14 years of age were randomly assigned to CIFFTA or individual treatment as usual (ITAU) showed that:

- CIFFTA had significantly higher retention (83%) than the comparison condition (71%), odds ratio = 2.05, $p = .036$.
- Youth in both conditions had significant reductions in child- and parent-reported externalizing and internalizing behaviors and no significant differences between conditions.
- Parents in CIFFTA reported significantly greater reductions in family conflict, $d = 0.38$, $p = .025$, than in the comparison condition.
- In CIFFTA, children of less acculturated Latine parents showed more improvement than the children of more acculturated parents.

CIFFTA's superior impact on retention and reduction of family conflict was a significant finding even though both conditions show treatment effects on youth behavior problems. This evidence of differential effects depending on cultural

> values and behaviors may have strong implications for the field of Latine psychology, family treatment, and the tailoring that may be necessary when working with diverse Latine clients.

Following its record of testing in the research arena with diverse populations, CIFFTA was selected for implementation by community agencies in the South Florida area. This allowed us to evaluate the effectiveness of implementing CIFFTA for the treatment of 232 Latine and Black youth and families in community settings (Mena et al., 2024b). Utilization of services offered, changes in youth presenting problems, and family functioning were used to evaluate the program. As we discuss in Chapters 9 and 10, there are many factors that determine whether an EBT is successfully transported to the community, and there is as much of a need for an *evidence-based approach to implementation and sustainability* as there is for EBTs.

In the community setting for this program evaluation, care coordinators and natural helpers (*promotoras*) formed part of the team. After they learned about what an intervention such as CIFFTA has to offer youth and families, they were able to reach parts of the community that are typically highly underserved and that do not always trust community programs. Natural Helpers are often members of the community who were connected and trusted long before the EBT was offered. The evaluation results showed a program with great retention of families as shown by the percentage of families completing treatment, strong participation in the program as shown by number of sessions (average of 15 sessions) received per family, improvement in youth behavioral and emotional presenting problems, and improvements in family functioning.

Mena et al. (2024b) Study Details

This project that included 232 Latine and Black youth and families, allowed us to evaluate the effectiveness of implementing CIFFTA in community settings. Findings revealed that:

- Adolescents reported a significant reduction in symptoms of *depression* ($N = 147, Z = -3.63, p < .001$).
- Adolescents reported a significant reduction in symptoms of *anxiety* ($N = 147, Z = -3.01, p = .003$).

- Caregivers reported significantly lower *overall adolescent difficulties* ($N = 147, Z = -4.45, p < .001$) as did the adolescents ($N = 147, Z = -5.06, p < .001$).
- Caregivers reported a statistically significant reduction in *family conflict* ($N = 146, Z = -4.68, p < .001$) and a significant increase in *family cohesion* ($N = 145, Z = -2.53, p = .011$).
- Caregivers reported a statistically significant reduction in *parental stress* ($N = 145, Z = -3.69, p < .001$).
- Caregivers reported a significant decrease in *frustration with their relationships with their children* ($N = 146, Z = -4.40, p < .001$), improved *parent–adolescent communication* ($N = 147, Z = -3.43, p < .001$), and improved *confidence in parenting* ($N = 146, Z = -2.93, p = .003$).

SUMMARY

In this chapter, we have argued for the important role that EBTs can play in optimally serving Latine youth and families, pitfalls that must be avoided, and why we believe that CIFFTA offers a unique set of tools that can be particularly effective with this population. We gave the reader a feel for CIFFTA's unique interventions and how it creates synergy between the three components to lead to more effective treatment. Finally, we provided some evidence to show that a therapy that seeks to integrate cultural and established therapy mechanisms can be tested in rigorous randomized trials and show its efficacy and effectiveness with diverse and complex problems.

The experience of these trials has led to the development of expertise in training clinicians to implement family-based interventions and the development of innovative training platforms (see Chapter 9). Most of the work on CIFFTA has been done with Latine youth and families, but more recent implementations of CIFFTA with African American and Haitian youth are leading to the articulation of unique stressors that can be considered for tailoring within the CIFFTA framework (see Chapter 10). Our CIFFTA team has dozens of published articles, book chapters, and treatment guides focusing on treatment outcomes, family interventions, cultural competence, the training of family therapists, and the real-world problems of implementing EBTs.

2

The Latine Experience

Unique Stressors, Resilience, and Tools for Systematic Assessment

with Richard C. Cervantes

> Millions of people migrate each year. They do it alone or in organized aggregates, by their own decision or forced by decisions of others or by natural cataclysms, carrying with them truckloads of household items or a bundle of essentials. They travel on a luxury ocean liner or crammed in the bodega of a sampan, are received with press conferences, or sneak in under barbed wire borders by night. They look forward with hope or backward with fear. They belong to a culture in which high geographic mobility is the rule and count on skills to deal with the process of migration, or they have been raised in a highly sedentary culture in which uprooting means near-catastrophe. They are thoroughly familiar with, or completely ignorant of, their situation on arrival, the language and customs of the new place, the people, the dwelling situation, the work they are going to have. One way or another, countless numbers of people manage to break away from their basic support networks, sever ties with places and people, and transplant their home base, their nest, their life projects, their dreams, their ghosts.
>
> —Carlos Sluzki (1979)

These words by Carlos Sluzki are a powerful and poetic description of the range of experiences and emotions that we encounter in the lives of many different groups of immigrants and their descendants. They are a mix of extraordinary hope, unspeakable despair, and an overpowering sense of loss. Some families who have been in the United States for generations carry the life experiences and the unfulfilled hopes

---

Richard C. Cervantes, PhD, Research Director, Behavioral Assessment, Inc., Los Angeles, California.

of their predecessors. Sluzki's words should open the eyes and heart of the therapist who wishes to truly connect with the realities of diverse Latine families.

In this chapter, we highlight unique experiences and stressors that have been identified in the field of Latine psychology and explain how these impact adolescent and family well-being. These stressful life events often require making highly consequential decisions related to starting a new branch of the family tree in a foreign country. They include committing to a country that may not always appear to welcome you and your family, no matter how many generations your family has been in the country. It includes "accepting" that you and your family may struggle through complex processes that involve acculturation stress, economic stressors due to loss of occupational status, traumatic immigration experiences, and immigration-related family member separations. You may dread that your children might lose the beauty of their culture of origin because they *must* master the skills needed to succeed in the new host culture. It means using the hardships our ancestors went through to get to the United States to give our lives meaning and form the foundation of our resilience.

These client experiences directly impact your work with Latine youth and families. Culture and immigration-related characteristics may contribute to family-level risk factors as well as the development of family protective and resiliency processes. These unique experiences contribute to presenting problems, and can negatively impact child and adolescent development, family relationships and the fulfillment of key roles, family life cycle milestones, help-seeking behavior and treatment utilization, and therapy processes and outcomes. In this chapter we expand on these experiences and share a set of tools that can help you to identify and measure stressors faced by Latine youth and families. The measurement of these stress and resiliency profiles of Latine families can be key to successful case formulation and treatment planning. By making these processes central to the work, the treatment becomes more ecologically valid and increases its engagement, credibility, retention, and outcomes. The ease with which the therapist can identify with and communicate about these complex issues can contribute to enhanced client responses to treatment.

SEGMENTED MIGRATION AND IMMIGRATION-RELATED PARENT–CHILD SEPARATIONS

One of the clearest examples of how migration-related experiences can impact family processes and youth symptoms is when youth and caregivers are separated during the immigration experience (Mitrani et al., 2004; Suárez-Orozco & Suárez-Orozco, 2001). An exploration of these migration stories told uniquely by adolescents and caregivers shows how consequential this process can be for each of them. During treatment, we were able to link these separations to disruptions in key family processes such as relationship quality and parenting (Mitrani et al., 2004), to adolescent functioning (Santa-Maria & Cornille, 2007; Suárez-Orozco et al., 2010) and to adolescent depression (Mena et al., 2023).

There are many reasons for extended parent–child separations. Some do not involve the migration process at all (e.g., parent military service, incarceration of a parent, having a child live with extended family as a way of removing them from a noxious neighborhood), but here we will focus on those separations due to migration. This is most often seen when family members, specifically mothers and children, immigrate separately to the United States. One commonly occurring pattern involves women who have initiated their family's "stepwise" migration to the United States (Donato, 2010). This is different from the earlier patterns in which males took that first step to establish a beachhead in the United States, and mothers and children stayed together. Because there are more families headed by women, it is quite common to find women who lead the migration process, leaving children with extended family members in their country of origin and reuniting with them years later (Falicov, 2017). It is common that during the separation phase, children often deepen their relationship with their surrogate caregivers (e.g., grandmother). When reunification finally takes place, often 5–10 years later, the youth experience a second separation, this time from their surrogate figure (Suárez-Orozco et al., 2010). The reunification period is a difficult one because the expectation is that the family will be whole and happy when the long-awaited day arrives. The family is unprepared for the powerful feelings that are predictable, especially when the reasons and consequences of the separation are never fully processed by the family.

Mitrani et al. (2004) report the following powerful family processes that can occur in separated families, and which are the types of reactions a competent family therapist must be prepared to identify and work on:

- The child has strong feelings of abandonment and resentment but also feels guilt for having those negative feelings.
- The child experiences dual loyalties to the mother with whom they are reuniting versus the primary surrogate caretaker (often grandmother) to whom they became strongly attached during the separation but are now leaving behind.

- The family believes that the emergence of strong negative emotions is hurtful, disrespectful, and must be avoided.
- The mother may experience dual loyalties to new relationships (e.g., new partner and new children) and the reunited child(ren).
- Parenting behavior may be incongruent with the child's age as the parent attempts to treat the child as if time had not passed.

Within our program of research, Mena et al. (2023) investigated 163 Latine adolescents (64% males and 36% female) who were seeking treatment for substance use and related issues. The backgrounds of these adolescents' Latine parents were heterogeneous, but mainly from the Caribbean and Central and South America. Sixty-three percent of this specific sample of Latine youth had been born in the United States and had not experienced an immigration-related separation. However, 21% of the participants had experienced an immigration-related separation. For those adolescents who had experienced such a stressful separation from their mother, the average age at which the separation occurred was 7 years (SD = 4.6 years), and the average length of separation was over three and a half years (45.6 months) with a median of 24 months. Interestingly, when we compared immigration and nonimmigration-related separations, we found immigration-related separations to be longer, showing the difficulty with reunification once this type of separation is initiated.

One of the more interesting findings of this investigation is that the total time separated from the mother had a more clear-cut impact on the female than on the male adolescents. For girls only, longer separations were associated with more self-reported symptoms of internalizing disorders, particularly depression. Our findings on the relationship between adolescent internalizing disorders, immigration-related separations, total time separated, and gender have implications for our understanding of the youth and family impact that can be found in families at the time of reunification, years after the separation began.

ACCULTURATION-RELATED CHANGES WITHIN INDIVIDUALS AND FAMILIES

Acculturation, as a source of stress, can also have a substantial impact on a family's well-being. Acculturation is a core experiential process that affects individuals and families when they enter a new context that is dominated by a different culture. Berry (1992) defines acculturation as a complex process that results from contact between two or more autonomous cultural groups and their individual members. Acculturation often involves changes in a person's values and behavioral repertoire. These cultural, psychological, and behavioral changes sometimes take years and even generations to fully unfold. People show different profiles of acculturation, and they can vary in the degree to which they adapt (Berry, 2005). Rudmin (2009) recommends that (1) acculturation be defined as second-culture acquisition; (2) acculturative motivations, learning, and changes be conceived, measured, and sometimes studied independently of mental health issues; (3) bidimensional measures that separately assess Hispanicism and Americanism be used because unidimensional measures of "high" or "low" acculturation are inadequate; and (4) the impact of socioeconomic status and discrimination always be considered. Previous unidimensional models that suggested that the culture of origin is simply *replaced* by new cultural elements failed to account for individuals who kept new *and* old cultural elements active in their daily lives (Sam & Berry, 2010). Some individuals can show a *bicultural* profile where they display elements of both cultures, an *assimilation* profile where they display mostly elements of the new host culture, a *separation* profile where they display mostly the old cultural elements, and a less commonly found *marginalization* profile where they shun elements of both cultures.

In addition to looking at the different ways in which an individual can endorse either or both the culture of origin and the host culture, it is also important to distinguish different domains for acculturation processes. Schwartz et al. (2010) describe acculturation as operating within the domains of practices, values, and identifications. *Practices* can include such things as language use, media preferences, and choice of friends. One of the most used proxies or indicators of acculturation in Latines is language used at home or fluency in English and Spanish. *Values* can include such things as individualism, collectivism, and familism. Values are often conveyed in covert ways and are not always explicitly discussed or acknowledged. Cultural *identifications* refer to how one identifies in terms of nationality and ethnicity. As Schwartz et al. (2014) highlight, it is important to understand that acculturation profiles can look different in each of the domains, and these differences can have important treatment implications.

When we expand beyond the individual to take the entire family as the unit of analysis, the acculturation picture *becomes even more complex and interesting* because different family members tend to acculturate to different degrees and at different rates. When some family members (e.g., adolescents) are changing rapidly while others (for example, caregivers) are changing slowly or not at all, the discrepancy or gap between the values and behavior profiles of different family members becomes an additional stressor and can become a source of family conflict. Differences that are expected between generations (e.g., parent–child differences due to age) are multiplied when the older generation is also adhering to different culture-related values (from the country and culture of origin) than the more acculturated youth. In effect, generational and cultural discrepancies combine to create increased distance between family members. This cannot be said to lead inevitably to conflict, but it can be an added source of stress that may be handled well or poorly.

THE ACCULTURATION PARADOX

A surprising but consistent finding in the field is that recent Latine immigrants often show fewer signs of poor mental health and substance misuse than non-Latine Whites and Latines who have been in the United States for longer periods of time. The symptoms of recent immigrants are lower than would be expected given their negatively impacted socioeconomic status, exposure to immigration stress, social stress, ill-defined legal status, and acculturation demands. Considerable research has shown that the positive mental health status of Latines tends to erode with time spent in the United States (Marks et al., 2014).

Why would Latines who have been in the United States much longer, who are more adapted to the new surroundings, and who are mastering the language show more signs of mental health and substance use difficulties? One hypothesis is that over time, immigrants gain access to an entirely new set of opportunities, norms, and habits, some of which are risky and may include behaviors that had been more restricted in the country of origin. Another hypothesis focuses on the erosion of the traditional values toward family, a strong sense of cultural identity, and extended family support that had served as protective factors to promote resilience. Negative changes observed in mental health status may be linked to the erosion of family and culture-related resilience factors and changes in what had been protective family processes, including traditional parenting (Ríos-Ellis et al., 2005; Santisteban et al., 2012). Finally, there is the power of broken hopes and dreams—the realization that prosperity does not come as easily as had been hoped, that hardship may be long term, and that one is restricted to a tiny apartment that is in a neighborhood that is too dangerous to allow the children to go out and play. These can be disheartening. And the disappointment is amplified when one perceives that society may be working against the success of people like themselves. It recalls the powerful poem by Langston Hughes called "Harlem," also known as "Dreams Deferred" (Hughes, 1994).

ACCULTURATION STRESS

Berry (1991) described "acculturation stress" as the stress that can result from one's culture of origin interacting with host culture values, attitudes, customs, and behaviors. Individuals and families from one cultural orientation who are constantly being exposed to novel and challenging values, events, and situations require constant psychological and behavioral adjustments. Any significant adjustment (e.g., a new language, a new system, the challenges of economic advancement, a new set of rules and norms for raising children and for marital relationships) can create stress in an individual and the family. Exposure to racial or ethnic discrimination (such as anti-immigrant messages) can constitute additional sources of daily stress that may require an individual or family to adjust their living circumstances, choice of where to work, or choice of school to bring a sense of personal or familial safety, balance, and harmony (Romero & Roberts, 2003). The experience of marginalization can lead an individual to realize they are a "minority" for the first time. Stress related to the acculturation process has been linked to increased substance use (Unger et al., 2014), alcohol consumption (Caetano et al., 2007), cigarette smoking (Detjen et al., 2007), and HIV risk (Amaro et al., 2002). When individuals and families lack internal or social resources to cope with acculturation stress, an imbalance can occur that can overwhelm the ability to cope effectively.

The acculturation stress process itself may best be framed within a stressful life-events paradigm (Rudmin, 2009). In this paradigm social organization plays a significant role in the origins and consequences of stressful life experiences (Aneshensel, 1992). Lazarus and Folkman (1984) articulated the concept of stress appraisal, which is the subjective psychological reaction to stressful events. Negatively appraised stressor events related to acculturation can be important antecedents for mental health problems in both adults and children (Cervantes et al., 1991; Cortes et al., 1994; Vega & Gil, 1998). Social support and traditional values tend to erode over time and with greater exposure to American society. Risk factors such as increases in marital instability, low educational attainment, increased experimentation with drugs and alcohol, and changes in emotional support structures and gender roles all become more prevalent among Latines as they spend more time in the United States. Cervantes has conducted a series of research studies among both Latine youth and adults and identified a complex set of culturally related stressor experiences that are strongly correlated with poor mental health and behavioral health problems including depression and self-harm, internalizing/externalizing behavior problems, and substance use (Cervantes et al., 2012, 2014; Berger Cardoso et al., 2016).

As mentioned above, acculturation-related stress takes on a unique form when we expand our focus from the individual to family relationships and we note that practices, rituals, values, beliefs, and identifications change at different rates within a family. Over time, the family members may no longer share the values and worldviews that formed a type of glue that held a family together. It is often the case that parents will feel that the youngsters are endorsing "problematic" values and beliefs such as speaking their minds in all situations, challenging authority, and having more relaxed ideas about sexuality and substance use. In addition, there may be a feeling that kids are forgetting or rejecting the culture and values that define the country of origin. Children can be blamed for disrespecting the culture of origin and failing to appreciate its importance.

When these discrepancies are found within families, they are not always occurring between kids and parents. Different rates of the acculturation process can create stress between partners, spouses, and extended family who may be involved in caregiving. Culture-related family and couples' conflicts, as well as acculturation gaps between parents and children have been identified as core acculturation stress constructs (Cervantes et al., 2015). Fortunately, this is a process that is right in the wheelhouse of a culturally informed family therapist and successfully working through these issues can make a powerful difference in the quality of family relationships (Santisteban et al., 2013).

MINORITY STRESS

An important model for working with individuals and groups that tend to be highly marginalized is the Minority Stress Model (Meyer, 2003; Goldbach & Gibbs, 2015). Stress typically occurs when external conditions and demands exceed the resources that the individual has available to them to endure the demands (Dohrenwend, 2000). Among these stressors are discrete events as well as chronic and long-standing conditions related to social structures and policies that invalidate rather than support a person's worldview and lifestyle. Minority Stress can be thought of as the excess stress that comes from belonging to a stigmatized social category or minority position. That is, stress is attributable to more than any individual deficit but is found in the interaction of individuals in an unwelcoming social and political context. In addition to run-of-the-mill stress, the minority person experiences additional forms of stress when the dominant culture and its social structures and norms do not reflect the worldview, beliefs, and expectations of the minority group (Cyrus, 2017; Meyer, 2003).

Myers (2003) describes *distal stressors* as those that are external conditions and forces. Distal stressors can include discrimination, prejudice, and stereotypes. More *proximal stressors* include things that are internalized in the individual and can include internalized homophobia, expectations of rejection, and concealment. The role that Minority Stress can play in promoting negative physical and mental health outcomes has been studied in relationship to eating disorders (Convertino et al., 2021), substance use (Goldbach et al., 2015), and other presenting problems. Cyrus (2017) has written about individuals such as LGBTQ+ people of color who fit the label of *multiple minorities* and may be multiply marginalized.

RECEPTION IN THE HOST COUNTRY

Escalating anti-immigrant sentiments and policies can negatively impact youth and family development. These efforts put many Latine children who are U.S. citizens by birth, in a state of constant vigilance about having one or more of family members deported. Indeed, most Latine children (52%) are U.S.-born to foreign-born parent(s), most commonly from Mexico. Over 3.2 million second-generation Latine children are threatened indirectly by deportation policies because they have at least one parent who is unauthorized to work or reside in the United States in what has been called a *mixed-status* family (Fry & Passel, 2009). When ethnic minority migrants experience discrimination, the result is often what Rumbaut (2008) has termed *reactive ethnicity*. Reactive ethnicity refers to holding even more strongly onto one's cultural heritage and resisting adoption of the receiving culture. In other words, discrimination may encourage ethnic minority families and their descendants to remain *separated* from the mainstream host/receiving culture (Schwartz & Unger, 2010). This response can be perceived by people of the dominant culture (including culturally insensitive teachers, therapists, and case workers) as a simple refusal to integrate because they are unaware of the systemic forces pushing individuals in the direction of separation.

PLACING RESILIENCE ON THE RADAR SCREEN ALONG WITH RISK

Although acculturation and immigration-related stress can result in a variety of mental health concerns, most families exhibit resilience of various forms. *Resilience* is defined as the capacity to overcome adversity and even use the adversity to promote growth. As you work with families, you will want to look for protective factors and acknowledge that protective factors can be independent of risk factors. For example, risk and protective factors can exist in the same family at the same time. Indeed, true protective effects are most obvious when negative consequences expected due to risk, do not emerge. Think of the protection that hurricane shutters offer as a hurricane surrounds a home. Or think of the protection that seat belts or football helmets offer in the face of risk factors such as auto accidents or head-to-head collisions during a football game. The adverse effects that would be expected due to the collisions are diminished by the existence of the protective mechanisms. You are not eliminating or avoiding the risk factor, you are avoiding the negative consequence that typically results from the risk factor. One of the most important reasons for working with families is that you can mobilize and enhance the protective processes (e.g., support, validation, guidance) that can reduce the adverse effects on a youth who is facing marginalization, racism, and neighborhoods in which there is easy access to drugs.

For these reasons, resilience has become an important concept in developmental science and in the field of mental health over recent decades. Resilience involves dynamic processes fostering positive adaptation in the context of significant life stressors (Masten & Cicchetti, 2016). *Family resilience* refers to the capacity of the family as a functional system to overcome adversity (Walsh, 2016). Strengthening the family's skills and strategies in mastering immediate challenges also increases its resourcefulness in meeting future life challenges. In a recent study we were successful in identifying and linking new constructs of Latine family resilience processes within Walsh's family resilience framework (Cervantes & Santisteban, 2016). Studies focused on a protective factor known as *familismo* (an orientation toward family) find favorable psychosocial results for Latine children (Calderón-Tena et al., 2011; Morcillo et al., 2011), and adolescents (Germán et al., 2009; Marsiglia et al., 2009). Incorporating Latine family values into early intervention and prevention programs can prevent the erosion of traditional family protective factors (Castro & Alarcón, 2002).

Because of the central role of *familism* (or *familismo*) in Latine families, it is worth going more in depth into this topic. Emphasis on family life is a central core value to most Latines and serves as a key factor in family resiliency. The concept of familism is a belief in the centrality of family. It highlights family loyalty, obligation, interdependence over independence, and cooperation over competition (Ho et al., 2004). Familism, along with several other important Latine cultural values (i.e., *simpatia,* power distance, personal space, present time orientation, traditional gender roles) may impact health outcomes and can change during the acculturation process (Gallo et al., 2009). Familism has been linked to family stability, better physical health behaviors, higher likelihood of seeking medical help, better psychological health, and lower perceived burden of stress (Bermudez & Mancini, 2013). Familism and the highly involved parenting practices that were shown to be associated with familism have been linked to fewer behavior problems in the children (Santisteban et al., 2012). Because families that reported higher familism tended to be more highly involved parents and had youth with fewer behavior problems, the authors warn against prematurely labeling these parents as "enmeshed and over-involved." In these families a continuing connection to the culture of origin appeared to be protective. The issue of distance, whether very close or very distant, should not be prematurely judged as adaptive or maladaptive until the reasons for it (e.g., kids staying away from a parent who is misusing substances) and/or the impact on well-being (e.g., high involvement leading to more safety in risky neighborhood) are fully understood.

Taken together, there is a large and growing body of research demonstrating that many individuals and families are subject to a range of acculturation-based, immigration-based, and minority-related stressors. These stressors can accumulate, disrupt family systems and support, and negatively impact behavioral health. When clinicians are unaware of the impact of these stressors, or when they choose to avoid directly addressing these stressors, clients may feel that therapy and therapists are oblivious to the real struggles of the family. Standardized methods for assessing acculturation and immigration stress, as well as culturally based resilience (e.g., strong *familismo*), can play a significant role in preparing the provider to be more effective by facilitating treatment planning.

ADVANCES IN THE ASSESSMENT OF ACCULTURATION AND STRESS

If constructs such as acculturation, acculturation stress, and immigration-related stress are going to be useful, it is helpful to have tools available for measuring these complex conditions. In the next sections we present major advances in the measurement of these constructs. These have been invaluable because we can not only quickly assess the profile of an individual but also the differences between family members. The use of the Hispanic Stress Inventory–2 (HSI-2; Cervantes et al., 2016) for adults and the Hispanic Stress Inventory—Adolescent Version (HSI-A; Cervantes et al., 2011) for youth have yielded benefits to therapists during case formulation, treatment planning, and treatment tailoring. The ability to measure specific contexts of acculturation stress that are not commonly assessed during an intake session can be helpful to researchers, counselors, and clients alike. Prior to the development of the HSI, HSI-A, and HSI-2, most clinicians relied on their own personal cultural backgrounds or notions of acculturation stress. There were no standardized assessment tools to provide a full assessment of the various contexts in which acculturation and immigration-related stressors occurred.

Measuring Acculturation

Assessment of acculturation can include measuring (1) the degree to which a client has acquired aspects of the new culture (e.g., American culture), (2) the degree to which the client maintains their own language and cultural orientation, and (3) the client's ability to easily function in both the new culture and culture of origin (i.e., bicultural). Because a Latine youth and family member that self-reports being highly "Americanized" may react differently to an intervention than a youth or family member that reports being highly "Hispanic" (Santisteban et al., 2022), this type of measure can guide treatment planning and help explain client responses to treatment. In our 2022 research, these measures helped us answer the research question "what worked best for whom?"

The different acculturation profiles described by Sam and Berry (2010) remind us that we should measure how an individual endorses values, practices, and identifications as it relates to the country of origin *and* to the new host country. Is the individual acquiring new values, beliefs, and behaviors while also holding onto the existing values, beliefs, and behaviors? Can an individual enjoy both types of food, use both languages comfortably, dance to music from both cultures, and is that ability helping the individual feel more comfortable in many settings and in connecting with younger peers as well as with older generation family members? Are there pressures pushing the individual to "choose" one way of being? A measure should be able to show the individual's endorsement of both dimensions (in this case what has been called Americanism and Hispanicism) separately and independently. We will leave for another day an attempt to unpack the term *Americanism* given that U.S. culture has itself already been significantly impacted by Latine culture as evident in the popularity of tacos, burritos, Goya foods, bicultural performers, salsa, merengue and reggaeton music, and Cinco de Mayo celebrations.

Measuring Acculturation Stress

Hispanic Stress Inventory—Adolescent Version

Cervantes and colleagues (Cervantes et al., 2011, 2012) have a program of instrument development that has contributed several tools for measuring stress in Latine populations. Evaluating stress in Latine youth, the HSI-A measures eight unique domains of stress related to acculturation stress. Some domains are strongly associated with processes related directly to being a Latine in the United States (e.g., immigration stress, acculturation stress, and family economic stress). Others tap into stress at the family level (acculturation gap stress between parent and youth, family drug and legal stress, family-related immigration stress). Finally, other subscales measure stressful experiences related to socioeconomic disadvantage (Evans & Kim, 2007) such as community safety and gang stress, and discrimination. Not coincidentally, many of the categories that are assessed using this tool match those outlined in the stress and family process literature presented earlier in the chapter.

The practical value of the HSI-A can be seen in the research linking these stressors to depression (Cervantes et al., 2014), suicide-related behavior and ideation (Cervantes et al., 2014), and risky substance use behaviors (Berger Cardoso et al., 2016). In a study using the HSI-A, Latine youth who used alcohol had significantly higher HSI-A scores across five domains: acculturation gap, community gang, family economic, discrimination, and family drug-related stress (Goldbach et al., 2015). Each of these studies has shown high scale scores measured by the HSI-A to be linked to a variety of negative mental health or substance use outcomes in youth.

In clinical settings, acculturation stress and specific "contexts" of stress such as families, are critical areas for inquiry during the early assessment and treatment planning phases (Cervantes, 2017). The HSI-A can screen for culturally based stressors such as acculturation gaps, family immigration stress, gang-related stress and discrimination stress, and other relationally and contextually formulated domains of stress. As such, culturally informed early screening and assessment can prove beneficial to school personnel, as well as to trained clinicians who desire more relevant diagnostic information that can inform the treatment planning process. Family therapists can also have a more comprehensive and complete family case formulation when considering the role of acculturation stress. Table 2.1 includes subscales from the HSI-A and sample items.

Each of the subscales measures an independent area of acculturation stress with a unique set of items. A stress appraisal scoring system is used where the client is asked to endorse whether a particular stress

TABLE 2.1. Sample HSI-A Subscales and Item Content

Subscales	Question
Acculturation-Gap Stress	My parents want me to maintain customs and traditions from our home country.
Culture and Educational Stress	Teachers think I am cheating when I am speaking Spanish.
Immigration-Related Stress	I had to leave family members behind in my home country.
Community and Gang-Related Stress	There was a lot of pressure for me to get involved in gangs.
Discrimination Stress	Students made racist comments about me.
Family- and Drug-Related Stress	A family member had a drug problem.
Family Immigration Stress	Family members were afraid of getting caught by immigration officials.
Family Economic Stress	My family had problems paying rent.

event was experienced in the past year, and then using a 5-point Likert-type scale, to indicate how "stressful" the event was. Using standardized scores for each subscale provides the clinician with an assessment of high and low stress factors for the individual client. Using critical item analysis, the clinician can review each endorsed item and that stressor or traumatic event can be used in further clinical inquiry, integrated into a case formulation and can be flagged to be addressed by the clinician in treatment.

Hispanic Stress Inventory–2—Adult Version

An original version of the adult Hispanic Stress Inventory (HSI; Cervantes et al., 1991) was revised to account for demographic and political shifts affecting Latine immigrants and later-generation Latines in the United States (Cervantes et al., 2016). Data collected in Los Angeles, El Paso, Miami, and Boston ensured good representation of the diverse issues present in different Latine groups across the United States. The immigrant version of the HSI-2—Adult Version includes 10 stress subscales, while the U.S.-born version includes 6 stress subscales. The revised HSI-2 highlights many of the changes that have occurred since the development of the original HSI and offers a deeper and more refined assessment of the subtle areas in which cultural stressors appear and impact wide cross sections of Latine adults, contemporary areas for clinical assessment and treatment planning.

Let's look at some examples of the significance of scores. A high HSI-2 score on the Pre-Migration subscale can flag the types of important life experiences that occurred in the life of an immigrant client who may otherwise not have an opportunity to share these traumatic experiences that occurred *prior to migration*. Witnessing violence, experiences of extreme levels of economic deprivation, and other in-transit migration traumas and stressors (e.g., physical violence and rape) can be unresolved and serve as underlying causes of depression, anxiety, and posttraumatic stress disorder symptomatology. They may also explain and open the door to a discussion of the sadness, anxiety, and even guilt clients experience knowing that family members who stayed behind continue to experience these conditions.

Similarly, high scores on the HSI-2 Language Stress scores can be related to elevated anxiety and depression (Cervantes et al., 2018). Clients with high scores in this HSI-2 domain may have more limited access to community services and can benefit from English as a second language classes or academic tutoring services. This type of recommendation can become part of the case formulation and treatment plan. Additionally, for clinicians using DSM-5 (APA, 2013), certain *cultural formulations* can be aided by using the HSI-2 to determine areas in which clients may be experiencing high levels of acculturation stress. This information is specifically important for addressing psychosocial stressors and cultural features of vulnerability and resilience, as identified by the Cultural Formulation Interview (CFI; American Psychiatric Association, 2013). Table 2.2 lists a sample of subscales and sample questions from

TABLE 2.2. HSI-2 Sample Subscales—Nonimmigrant Version and Item Content

Subscales	Question
Discrimination Stress	I have been discriminated against.
Marital Stress	I have felt that my spouse and I have not been able to communicate.
Health Stress	I could not pay for my medical care.
Family-Related Stress	I had serious arguments with family members.
Parental Stress	I have thought that my children used illegal drugs.
Occupation Stress	Others have been too worried about the amount and quality of work I do.
Unemployment and Economic Stress	I lost my job.

TABLE 2.3. HSI-2 Subscales—Immigrant Version and Item Content

Subscales (adds four different subscales)	Question
Immigration-Related Stress	My legal status has been a problem in getting a good job.
Marital Acculturation-Gap Stress	My spouse and I disagreed about going back to our home country.
Language-Related Stress	Not knowing English made it difficult to find a job.
Preimmigration Stress	I was forced to leave my home country due to poverty.

the HSI-2 Immigrant and Non-Immigrant Versions. Table 2.3 shows the immigrant version of the HSI-2 adds four different subscales.

HSI-A and HSI-2 scoring procedures and clinical profiles determine how high a particular subscale score may be for an individual client in comparison to norms. Using the HSI-2 as a pre- and posttreatment measure can also assist clinicians in determining where certain areas of acculturation stress have been reduced or eliminated. Lower posttreatment scores on the HSI-2 would indicate that (1) the source of a particular acculturation stress complex has been removed or eliminated from the individual's life, or (2) there is a set of strategies that have been mobilized in the therapeutic process to assist the client to achieve more effective coping with the stressors and thereby reduced subjective experience of stress. Recommendations for using the HSI-A and HSI-2 as part of the intake process were described in *A Guide for Conducting Cultural Assessment of Hispanic and Latine Clients* (Cervantes, 2017). This guide provides the clinician with a more open-ended, interview-type framework to assess acculturation stressors.

ASSESSMENT OF RESILIENCE/PROTECTIVE FACTORS IN LATINE CLIENTS

Family therapists increasingly seek to move beyond a focus on dysfunction and include strengths, resilience, and protective factors that can be enhanced even in the face of adversity and trauma (Walsh, 2016). Two promising resilience measures with a focus on Latines that are currently under development are worthy of mention here. These include the Hispanic Family Resilience Measure (HFRM; Cervantes & Santisteban, 2016) and the Hispanic Optimism Psychological Examination (HOPE;

Cervantes et al., 2023). The HFRM includes assessment of culturally specific resilience within a family context. HFRM core resilience themes include: Familism; Family Communication; Spirituality; Strong Ethnic Identity/Affiliations; Immigration Strategies and Legal Assistance; Traditional Latine Parenting; Education Enhancement Strategies; and Use of Community Resources Strategies. The groups of core themes and text segments from the transcripts were further abstracted into item stems. The first set of items captures the family's *current use* of resilience strategies, and a complementary set of items captures family *desire* to use the same set of strategies. A total of 8 HFRM sections are included in the final draft with 96 items assessing current family resilience and 82 items assessing desired use. The sections include Strategies for Discrimination (26 items), Strategies for Occupational/Financial Issues (22 items), Strategies for Marital and Couple Issues (22 items), Strategies for Parenting (24 items), Strategies for Immigration Issues (24 items), Strategies for Family Conflicts (26 items), Strategies for Managing Health (20 items), and Strategies for Language Issues (16 items). This HFRM continues to be developed with the hope that it will provide clinicians and counselors with another Latine-specific assessment to aid in the case formulation and treatment tailoring efforts.

The HOPE measure evolved from research on immigration and acculturation stress (Cervantes et al., 2023). Optimism has been shown to be a critical form of resilience, particularly among immigrants. The ability to measure and assess areas of personal optimism as a resilience resource is useful to the treatment process. The HOPE measure was informed by research on the HSI-2 and now includes three factorially derived subscales (Optimism for Family, Optimism for Personal Wellbeing/Freedom, Optimism for Economic Achievement) that are strongly related to overall health and behavioral health factors.

SUMMARY

This chapter highlighted major life experiences and stressors that Latine clients and families face during the process of migration, acculturation, and integration into the new host culture and community. We presented studies linking these stressors directly to different aspects of adolescent and family functioning. In the second part of the chapter, we focused on tools for the systematic assessment of these key processes, showing specific items and how family members can report on their impact on the family. Many families may never be aware of the links between the stressors and negative impacts on their well-being, until they respond to the questions posed in such as assessment. The inclusion of these conversations adds depth to the therapy process and makes treatment more ecologically valid. We also introduced the importance of resilience in the lives of Latine youth and families and the ways in which resilience can be considered and measured. As family therapists we must make sure to avoid focusing only on the stressors and dysfunction and miss the powerful processes that Latine families rely on to stay healthy in the face of great adversity.

3

Foundations of Effective Treatment of Latine Youth and Families

In this chapter we present advances regarding culture and adolescent and family treatment that we consider foundational to CIFFTA and more broadly to working effectively with Latine clients. We highlight the innovations of dedicated clinicians, theorists, and researchers that continue to impact effective treatment today. CIFFTA is an evidence-based approach, and we believe there is a great benefit to using all its components designed uniquely to create synergy. But even if you choose not to adopt CIFFTA in its full manualized form, we still encourage you to consider the utility and wisdom of the foundational work presented here.

CULTURE-RELATED FACTORS THAT AFFECT PROBLEM DEVELOPMENT, HELP-SEEKING, AND THERAPY PROCESSES

We begin by presenting findings related to culture-related values and worldviews that can shape problem development, treatment-seeking behavior, and treatment processes. Several models are useful in exploring these factors. For example, the values orientation method provides an anthropological perspective that complements the usual way we think about behavior patterns and worldviews. After discussing the values orientation theory, we present models and frameworks that guide individually oriented treatment with adolescents. We end the chapter with advances that are the foundation of contextual and family therapy. These include the highly influential Ecological Framework developed by Uri Bronfenbrenner. This framework is particularly important because it helps therapists to conceptualize both the adolescent and the family within a much larger set of contexts and influences (e.g., larger systems such as schools, the judicial system, cultural messaging, and structural inequities). By doing this, we can identify additional targets of change and contextual interactions we seek to enhance (e.g., effective parental advocacy in the school or juvenile justice systems).

Values Orientation Theory

Values Orientation Theory provides a framework for understanding values that are deeply ingrained and shape the way everyday activities, events, and relationships are interpreted and defined. Szapocznik et al. (1978) used the values orientations work conducted by Kluckhohn and Strodtbeck (1961) to better understand Latine families in treatment. Four basic values orientation postulated by Kluckhohn and Strodtbeck are presented here along with examples of their influence on therapy process.

The *Relational Orientation* dimension is particularly impactful from a family process and therapy perspective. It focuses on whether people favor (1) hierarchical (vertical relationships), (2) collateral (i.e., a more horizontal network) and/or (3) individualistic (i.e., emphasizing autonomy) relationships. Individuals endorsing a hierarchical orientation may be particularly open to a family-oriented therapy as compared to a peer group therapy or individually oriented therapy. A preference for vertical relationships may also be particularly compatible with one of the most cited Latine preferences, *familism*, which we discuss below.

A preference for hierarchical/vertical family relations can have implications for the emergence of disagreement and conflict resolution, which are key processes in family functioning. When parents view good family functioning as nonegalitarian and characterized by clear-cut levels of authority and obedience, they can perceive any type of open disagreements by an adolescent as disrespectful and unacceptable. Therapists must identify this situation to avoid prematurely asking adolescents to speak their mind in session in a way that the parents feel is disrespectful and undermining of their authority. This intervention may be seen by parents as making the problem worse, by encouraging what is perceived to be the dysfunctional behavior (e.g., disrespectful and challenging behavior). Furthermore, cultures that value harmony in relationships and *respeto* (respect) may make frequent use of conflict diffusion and avoid conflict emergence. These culture-related characteristics can impact therapeutic processes such as direct negotiation and problem solving between adolescents and parents. This does not mean that therapists must avoid open negotiation in therapy, but that they must first prepare the ground and have a deeper understanding of the family assumptions and orientations that may initially reject such an intervention.

The *Human Nature* orientation includes variants that may consider human nature as (1) good, (2) bad, or (3) neutral. An experienced family therapist who has worked with diverse clients will have worked with parents who see their misbehaving children as inherently "bad" or even described as "influenced by evil." This position is powerful and qualitatively different from parents who see behavior as problematic but perceive the child as inherently good. When the person is deemed to be the sole problem (particularly if they are seen as bad by nature), all responsibility for a problem is rigidly attributed to that one person while other family or relational contributions to the problem are minimized. This makes it that much more difficult for a therapist to expand the definition of the problem to a more systemic, relational, and contextual one. Family members may be less willing to accept the need to change family relationship patterns. It should not be surprising that many Afro-Caribbean families often attribute psychological symptoms to spiritual problems and therefore may be more likely to seek the counsel of a minister or spiritual leader. The mismatch between a family's perception of the "cause" of the problem (i.e., evil) and what a therapy has to offer, can contribute to difficulties in engagement of families into therapy (Santisteban & Szapocznik, 1994). A more complete understanding of this mismatch can help the therapist expand the family's view of the problem and solution.

The *Person–Nature Dimension* refers to the perceived relationship of people to natural phenomena with a range of (1) subjugation to nature, (2) harmony with nature, and (3) mastery over nature. Many Western models of therapy are founded on the value of mastery over nature (i.e., identifying and changing those characteristics that are problematic). Conversely, cultures that value acceptance over mastery may strive to help a person to accept rather than conquer a major health or mental health condition. Families that value acceptance of life difficulties and the will of a higher power may sometimes be mislabeled as passive and unmotivated. A client may say, "If this is God's will, I will accept it." A therapist must have the capacity to meet the family where they are at and then seek to negotiate the expansion of that perspective if it will contribute to their well-being.

What does accepting such a worldview of subjugation and acceptance and then expanding it look like? Perhaps it would look like processing with the client the old story of the man caught in torrential rains that caused the dam to break, flooding the valley, and trapping the man on top of the roof of his home. He prayed that God would miraculously rescue him. When a boat came by and invited him to come aboard, he declined, saying that God would rescue him. As the floodwaters continued to rise a helicopter flew by and lowered a rope ladder, but once again the man declined rescue, giving the same answer. When the man finally drowns and reaches the Gates of Heaven he yells, "God, I prayed and prayed! Why didn't you rescue me?" God looks him in the eye and says, "I sent you a boat and a helicopter. What more do you want?" Perhaps an expansion of an "acceptance" position would be that it may be God's will that the client accepts the help being sent to them to battle the present circumstances. *When Faith Meets Therapy,* a book cowritten by a religious leader and a therapist (Evans & Kaiser, 2022), serves as an example of integration and expansion in a way that removes stigma from all sides and has the potential to reach across the divide. We expand on this discussion because while we often describe Latines as highly spiritual and religious, we do not always think through the implications for our work. For many of the families we work with and for whom faith is a core component of their lives, it is imperative that we be prepared to create a bridge from faith to our therapeutic approach.

The *Time Orientation Dimension,* refers to the emphasis placed on a particular time in one's life, with a range of (1) present, (2) past, and (3) future. Zimbardo and Boyd (1999) call this variable *time perspective* and found it to be a valid and reliable individual difference variable. An understanding of the time orientation of our client has considerable value for the planning of interventions. A therapist implementing a prevention intervention (which is future oriented) may be more effective when working with a client that has a future orientation rather than with families that are present-oriented and focused on today's issues. A present-oriented family may find the intervention more relevant and acceptable if its short-term benefits are emphasized.

When working with someone who is present-oriented, we may consider whether a drug prevention program will be more effective when framed as an intervention that targets current behavior problems or that provides coaching to increase effective behavior rather than one designed to prevent future drug use. These types of adaptations are consistent with the concepts proposed by Sue and Zane (1987), in which they recommend that interventions with minorities should be made clearly relevant to the client's daily lives, and that the credibility of the interventions and the therapist are crucial. The perceived credibility of a therapy and the degree to which a proposed intervention makes sense to clients, has been shown to affect therapeutic outcomes (Constantino et al., 2018). It should be noted that socioeconomic conditions or environment may have much to do with a present orientation, such as when a family must struggle to survive day to day.

Familism

One of the characteristics most studied and written about in relation to families of diverse ethnic backgrounds is their emphasis on the family (e.g., nuclear, extended, and kinship networks) over the individual. Marín and Marín (1991) have shown how Latines often report higher levels of interdependence, conformity, loyalty, and readiness to sacrifice for the welfare of family members. Sabogal et al. (1987) have divided the construct of familism into three basic dimensions: (1) Family Obligations, (2) Perceived Support from the Family, and (3) Family as Referents. An understanding of how these values play out in families is essential to understanding how the family can be used as a resource in therapy. By investigating the relationship between acculturation and these core dimensions, the authors found that with greater acculturation came reductions in the endorsement of "Family Obligations" and "Family as Referents." They found that acculturation did not modify the extent to which individuals perceived "Support from the Family." That is, "Perceived Support from the Family" remained constant even among highly acculturated individuals. Interestingly, even though "Family as Referents" tended to decrease with acculturation, even acculturated Latines were significantly higher on this dimension than were White non-Latines. The value placed on the family can have powerful influences on the treatment processes because it can be cited as a central reason that motivates a client to change their maladaptive behaviors. That is, some individuals may be motivated to change not by consequences to themselves as individuals but by the potential negative or positive impact on the family and/or the family's reputation.

A therapist working with families consisting of multiple members with differing needs must be aware that there are benefits and pitfalls associated with any given orientation. Highly family-oriented families are very aware of and sensitive to each other's problems and needs and are often available for support. However, when taken to an extreme and implemented rigidly, families may not easily tolerate uniqueness so that those family members that do not "fit in" can be more readily ostracized and experience rejection. This may sometimes be the case with LGBTQ+ youth and other youth who chart a path that is not readily expected or accepted by the family. The lack of acceptance may be especially painful for a youth who endorses the importance of family closeness. A strength in families that are more individualistic, and that value autonomy may be that members learn how to be competent and independent at an earlier age. A challenge may be that in difficult times, family members are not available to support one another or may not even be aware of each other's emotional needs. Therapists must always be attentive to personal and cultural values and be careful not to undermine either the need for self-sufficiency or the reliance on other family members.

Traditionalism–Modernism

A related contribution to our thinking about the way culture can impact family and therapy processes comes from the work on the traditionalism–modernism continuum (Ramírez, 1999). More traditional lifestyles will have a much stronger emphasis on family ties, religion and spirituality, and cooperation. Conversely, a more modern lifestyle may include a stronger emphasis on individuality, competition, and individual achievement. The lifestyle will have repercussions on such important family matters as gender roles, sexuality, subservience to convention, religion, and the status of the elderly. In short, some key family members' behavior may be better understood by viewing them within the context of their position on the traditionalism–modernism continuum. Ramírez has developed an inventory that helps measure an individual's place on the continuum (Ramírez, 1999).

PILLARS OF ADOLESCENT THERAPY

In this section we present major contributions that are foundational to the individual interventions CIFFTA delivers to adolescents. The works contribute to how we conceptualize the relationships between behavior problems, adolescent motivation to change, the role of adolescent identities, and the types of skills that can make a difference in adolescent's lives.

Problem Behavior Syndrome

Co-occurring behavior problems are more the rule than the exception. This way of conceptualizing youth behavior suggests the possibility of a higher-order spectrum that includes such symptoms as substance use, risky sexual behavior, and delinquency from adolescence to young adulthood (Donovan & Jessor, 1985). It focuses on the interrelationships between symptoms *and* the need to identify underlying factors that may be fueling symptoms, driving problematic behaviors, or creating *generalized risk* and tendencies toward risk-taking (Palmer et al., 2009). The Problem Behavior Syndrome is used to describe individuals who tend to engage in an array of risk-taking behaviors and even more importantly, suggests that engaging in one behavior can increase the likelihood of engaging in another. The confluence of several risk-taking behaviors during the adolescent stage creates a concentrated threat that can disrupt healthy development and cause harm to the adolescent and others. Moffitt and Caspi (2001) describe *snares* as a set of problem behaviors such as leaving school prematurely, engaging in problem substance use, a criminal record, or incarceration, which trap the youth. These snares compromise the youth's ability to meet the challenges that emerge during the adolescent stage, challenges that must be met as part of a healthy transition into early adulthood.

Viewing behavior through the lens of a syndrome and snares makes it less attractive to consider treatments designed to address one symptom at a time. It becomes important to identify and treat the underlying condition(s) while working to identify less visible problems that are co-occurring and helping to maintain the entire symptom constellation. It helps when the clinician can identify how engaging in one problematic behavior may increase the likelihood of another. Although many of the models for the problem behavior syndrome tended to focus on individual characteristics that might underlie the syndrome, a more contextual approach to underlying conditions can be taken and used to guide treatment planning. The separate but related literature on *syndemics* has much in common with the problem behavior syndrome in its attention to the impact that presenting issues can have on each other. The problems have a compounding effect, serve to maintain each other, and create an even higher risk for some additional adverse outcomes. How often do you treat addiction in an adolescent without running into co-occurring depression or anxiety or emotion dysregulation or even problem peers that all serve to maintain the problem? When behaviors and symptoms are said to come together as a syndemic, the idea is that they are *interdependent* and that there is a *synergistic co-occurrence of multiple health problems* (Meyer, 2003).

Motivation Enhancement

A key to engaging an adolescent into treatment is to avoid becoming entangled in the type of power struggle that often emerges when someone other than the youth decides that the youth must change their behavior. The successful engagement of the youth and family members into services and into a partnership for change is one of the major tasks in the early phase of treatment. The challenge is to mobilize the adolescent's own interest in change, and to establish personal goals that emerge from their own vision of the future. Caregivers often initiate therapy, and it is often the case that adolescents are not on board with therapy and are not ready to change. If a therapist prematurely offers strategies for changing behavior (known as *change talk*), it may be a waste of time at best, and a way of creating resistance at worst. The therapist may simply be perceived as the person taking the place of the parent in the power struggle against the youth. Therapy will be most acceptable to the adolescent if it is perceived as focused on the personal and normative adolescent struggles they are experiencing and would like to work on. Motivation enhancement interventions help to mobilize those forces within the adolescent that can fuel change for the better so that the driving force is *within* them rather than external (i.e., parents, therapist, schools, and courts). Treatment is infinitely more effective when the adolescent provides the change goals and the reasons why the effort is worthwhile.

The outstanding work conducted by the developers of Motivational Interviewing (MI; Miller & Rollnick, 2023) provides a strong foundation for adolescent work. This intervention is designed to nurture the client's own creation of goals and reasons for behavior change rather than assume or impose reasons for change that feel alien to the client. Using MI, you can learn to explore the client's goals, perceptions, and experiences and encourage the emergence and amplification of discrepancies between present perspectives, behaviors, and long-term goals. Through acceptance and working through the ambivalence, the client becomes more engaged in the struggle toward self-definition and the relevance of therapy becomes clearer and more meaningful. Ambivalence can be defined as the state of having mixed feelings or contradictory ideas about something or someone, and it is a hallmark of the change process. Even after someone has initiated changes, ambivalence often re-emerges, and an important component of this work is amplifying and resolving ambivalence. A good clinician normalizes the experience of ambivalence using empathic and nonjudgmental responses. It is difficult to imagine how effective therapeutic work with an adolescent can take place without working on motivation enhancement.

A key to MI is the process of helping people move through the stages of change (Prochaska & DiClemente, 1992). The therapist learns to correctly identify the stage the client is in and to utilize the correct MI intervention that *fits* that stage. As we will show in later chapters that present the nuts and bolts of CIFFTA, we believe that accurate identification of current individual and family processes are important precursors to knowing what to do next. Too often we learn how to deliver an intervention without learning to discern the precise individual and family circumstance and moment that requires that specific intervention. To be effective a therapist must deliver the right intervention at the right time in a person's treatment. In the case of MI, a client that is at the *precontemplation stage* is not yet acknowledging that there is a problem behavior that needs to be changed (e.g., "I don't see what the big deal is that I like to drink and experiment with drugs, I am perfectly happy"). A set of interventions that recommends change strategies or the establishment of new goals is unlikely to succeed because it is not meeting the client where they find themselves. The client must first decide that there is a problem that is worth changing, before any plan for change is discussed.

Clients in the *contemplation stage* acknowledge that there is a problem, but they may not yet be ready or sure that they want to make a change (e.g., "I can see that my drinking and drug use may get me into trouble sometimes, but I don't see the need to go through all the work of changing at this time"). A client in a *preparation stage* is convinced that there is a problem and is getting ready to make a change. A client in the *action stage* is in the process of changing behavior. Finally, a person in the *maintenance stage* is working on maintaining the behavior change they have already accomplished. It is common for an individual to move forward in the stages and then seem to revert to a previous stage. The reader may want to make an honest assessment of the last time they tried to change a behavior that was deeply ingrained. Was it really a straight and steady line toward the desired behavior?

Therapy processes that elicit the client's own reason for change may be particularly helpful when working with minoritized clients because the client will provide reasons for change *that fit well with their worldviews and values*. For example, some clients who endorse familism and family obligations may incorporate family reasons for change, while others who are people of faith may incorporate spiritual reasons. The competent use of motivation enhancement strategies and techniques helps the therapist work alongside the client to evoke the client's motivations to change rather than become trapped in a blame game, a power struggle, or a cycle of generating one unmotivating reason for change after another.

Ethnic and Racial Identity

The early and late adolescent stages of development are characterized by a considerable amount of cognitive and physiological change and work on identity formation. The adolescent's development of an ethnic and racial identity is a complex and important adolescent process. Scholars who have contributed to the field have described the formation of ethnic and race identity within the context of developmental continuum from early childhood to middle childhood, to adolescence, and then to emerging adulthood (Umana-Taylor et al., 2014). This work focuses on important processes such as awareness of bias and social hierarchy, the internalization of cultural values, and the role of public regard. As we explored in Chapter 2, the well-being of a family is directly impacted by how their ethnic group is perceived and accepted by the host culture or context of reception. Individuals can experience poor treatment in their everyday interactions in major domains including school, peer network, workplace, neighborhoods, and due to language spoken, race, or class. This can be particularly painful and damaging to a youngster who has yet to fully develop an identity with which they are totally comfortable. For immigrant youth, there can be considerable differences between those youth who are born in the United States, those who immigrate to the United States during early childhood, and those who arrive later during adolescents or emerging adulthood. The emotional connection to their homeland and then the context of reception, whether pro or anti the ethnic and racial group to which the adolescent belongs, can also impact the pride or ambivalence experienced by the youth.

An influential way of thinking about the relationship between processes such as self-regulation and culture comes from the work of Yasui and Dishion (2007). They argue that culture and self-regulation cannot be thought of as independent and disconnected processes. Indeed, they argue that culture is endogenous to the family socialization process, and to the development of identity, strategies for self-regulation, coping strategies, and for meeting all the developmental challenges that are key during the adolescent stage.

Dialectical Behavioral Therapy Skills Training

Marsha Linehan's (1993, 2014a, 2014b, in press-a, in press-b) work stands as an extraordinary contribution to working with self-harm, substance use, and more generally shedding light on truly complex dynamics in the therapy relationship. Initially focused on the treatment of borderline personality disorder in adults, the rich detail and wisdom in Linehan's work makes it applicable to many clinical situations. Although CIFFTA does not use all the individually oriented strategies and approaches that are the foundations of Dialectical Behavior Therapy (DBT), there has been considerable work on the integration of family work with DBT (Fruzzetti et al., 2021). Furthermore, the psychoeducational skills training provides very powerful, practical ways of helping adolescents in treatment. We have found these skills helpful in the treatment of behavior problems, substance use, self-harm, and a general constellation of behaviors that resemble the borderline personality disorder profile (Santisteban et al., 2015). We do not believe that the skills component should be pulled out of a larger treatment and provided as a stand-alone component. In our work, skills were carefully integrated into the larger CIFFTA treatment approach. The complementary components of the larger treatment are needed to effectively address barriers to implementation of the skills and to the generalization of the skills to daily life.

Several of the skills are particularly effective with adolescents. *Emotion Regulation* focuses on teaching adolescents (1) how to identify their emotions and triggers to those emotions; (2) how to reduce their emotional vulnerability; and (3) how to react to negative emotions non-impulsively and in ways that lead to positive outcomes. The term *modulation* is preferred by many rather than regulation because it sounds less like "policing" of emotions and more like increasing or decreasing the volume/intensity of emotion much as we do with music (Fraenkel, 2023; Jurist, 2018). We tend to use the term *regulation* because it is more consistent with much of the literature. When adolescents who believe that their power comes from an emotional outburst, learn that they are in reality powerless when anyone can decide to set them off, they begin to see power in being less reactive to the whims of others. We often tell youth that they seem to walk around with a big red button on their chests and that anyone can set them off (and get them into trouble) just for fun. Learning emotion regulation skills helps them to disconnect the button and gain more control over their own actions and the subsequent consequences.

Interpersonal Effectiveness is another essential skill during the adolescent stage as they learn to identify emerging needs and to negotiate the satisfaction of those needs with powerful peers and adults. Interpersonal Effectiveness focuses on teaching adolescents (1) how to be more effective at identifying needs and selecting and reaching goals; (2) how to keep important relationships positive even as they ask that their needs be met; and (3) how to develop and maintain self-respect and feel good about oneself in challenging interpersonal contexts. These skills are essential when beginning intimate relationships, relationships with peers who try to normalize substance use and illegal behavior, and in family relationships that require new ways of relating to an emerging adult. In other words, these skills facilitate the complex work that comes with the adolescent developmental stage.

Finally, depending on the types of presenting issues the adolescents come to treatment with, *Crisis Management* and *Distress Tolerance* can also be powerful approaches. These skills are designed to assist clients in responding to intense events and negative emotional experiences. They teach participants how to manage their emotions and understand the link between emotions and thoughts. They also include relaxation and mindfulness strategies to assist in managing emotional and physical reactions to negative events.

As we will discuss later in this book, generalization of these learned skills to the daily lives of the adolescent is an important and powerful aspect of treatment. Family therapy sessions are the context in which adolescents can try on and practice the implementation of their new skills with family members and family therapists can facilitate this process in the service of healthier family functioning. Individual therapy sessions with the adolescent can also focus on the use of skills, particularly as they are applied with peers and teachers.

PILLARS OF CONTEXTUAL AND SYSTEMIC FAMILY THERAPY

In this section we present major contributions that are foundational to the family interventions CIFFTA delivers. The works contribute to how we conceptualize the adolescent and family within a larger set of contexts that create challenges and opportunities and that directly impact well-being, the strategies and techniques that can be used to bring about *in vivo* changes in family interactions, and ways of integrating culture-related knowledge and experiences into family work.

Ecological System Theory and the Adoption of a Contextual Approach

Adolescents do not live in a vacuum so a therapist must transition quickly from an individual perspective to one that considers the impact of the social systems that form the context of youth and family development and well-being. A contextual framework does not disregard or minimize the risk and protective factors that reside within the adolescent but expands to include those that reside within the family, school, and peer systems that are so influential in the adolescent's life. The framework also includes outer contexts including workplace pressures, and community and societal norms and policies that have ripple effects all the way down to the family and adolescent. Uri Bronfenbrenner's (2005) work highlights the processes that impact the emergence and maintenance of adolescent behaviors and how youth are intertwined with multiple systems and within complex systemic interactions (Cox et al., 2011). This framework is particularly helpful when therapists plan how, when, and where to intervene in the larger context. As we will show later in this book, the therapist has more options for intervening in a problem when the full set of contextual influences is considered.

The revised version of Bronfenbrenner's original theory (Bronfenbrenner, 2005; Rosa & Tudge, 2013; Tudge et al., 2009) emphasizes direct influences and encourages an emphasis on *proximal processes*. These proximal processes are the bidirectional interactions between the developing person (the adolescent in our work) and the other influential people within their environment (Bronfenbrenner, 2005). This provides a clearer focus on how adolescent well-being is impacted by specific individual adolescent characteristics that interact with characteristics of a specific context. This modification to the framework moves from a generic "trickle-down effect" to a more focused look at specific adolescent interactions with individuals in their ecology or what Koss and Vargas (1999) called the *activity settings* in which adolescents have unique interactions with key others.

For minoritized families, the framework also facilitates our look at the contextual/societal factors that contribute to difficulties of daily living. Societal policies, which are considered at the *macrosystem* level in the Bronfenbrenner model, are evident when undocumented families do not have the formal permission to be in the United States. Brietzke and Perreira (2017) used an ecological framework and qualitative interviews with first- and second-generation Latine youth living in North Carolina, to shed light on the stress, coping, and resilience factors that emerge in the context of accelerating enforcement activities aimed at undocumented immigrants. When families experience this disconnect with their country of residence and live in fear of being *seen,* they cannot avail themselves of many of the safeguards that most families take for granted. For example, victims of interpersonal violence may feel unable to report the violence for fear that the perpetrator or the victims themselves may be deported. Similarly, the family may feel the need to keep problem or illegal behavior by a child a secret to avoid deportation efforts. These are examples of contextual issues that directly and powerfully determine reactions to individual behaviors, within-family interactions, and family-therapist dynamics.

The Ecological Model can be used by experts in diverse fields to ensure that their specialized work does not stand alone but rather that it is conceptualized within the broader life context. Research has shown, for example, that in Latine families there is often strong adherence to a religious and spiritual life and this domain is often identified when investigating protective and resilience factors. Unfortunately, therapists often find it difficult to incorporate this area of work within their typical framework. Radillo (2007) in her beautifully delineated work on pastoral care, counseling, and therapy takes an ecological perspective. She argues for taking a "whole person" perspective and that pastoral counseling should carefully consider all the diverse factors that impact the person being cared for. Rather than allow the work in the spiritual domain to stand isolated, Radillo expands the perspective of her pastoral colleagues by offering a contextual and ecological perspective. She encourages a full embrace of what the social sciences have to offer, and the need to listen carefully to the lived experiences that include pain, discrimination, and oppression before prematurely offering solutions that do not validate that complexity. On the other side of the coin, when secular therapists struggle to acknowledge the importance and centrality of their clients' church and spiritual life, they would do well to follow Radillo's ecological perspective and better appreciate the spiritual protective functions that are key to their client's well-being. It would be a therapist's failure to disregard such a meaningful and powerful part of a client's life.

The original Bronfenbrenner model directs the therapist to assess how adaptively the family–school, family–peer, and family–health system mesosystems function. The well-being of the youth is promoted by healthy mesosystem interactions. For example, Hofstede's (1980) concept of power distance describes how some societies and diverse families favor marked power differentials. Here some people (i.e., doctors or highly educated specialists) or institutions (i.e., schools and medical settings) may be treated with the utmost respect, conformity, and deference. Families characterized by this orientation often expect hierarchical doctor–patient relationships (expert–patient) in which the doctor tells the patient what to do and the patient complies with little or no questioning. Treatment strategies that include multisystemic interventions (e.g., that attempt to help parents become advocates for the child within the school or juvenile justice systems) may be harder to implement because parents may feel intimidated or uncomfortable with requesting change from these systems. It is easy to label the behaviors resulting from this level of respect and awe of large institutions as passivity, dependence, and lack of motivation. To gain a full understanding of client values that impact "doctor–patient" relationships and the interactions between diverse parents and large institutions, requires that we carefully consider the influence of these contextual cultural influences and Hofstede's power distance orientation.

Koss-Chioino and Vargas (1999) made a major contribution to the field by bringing to life Bronfenbrenner's model and focusing on proximal processes, as they set the stage for Latine youth development and the role of culture in therapy. The authors use the contextual model to account for the "interaction among several factors: biopsychosocial processes (e.g., the information processing articulated by Martha Bernal and her colleagues); proximal processes (e.g., socialization by parents and significant caregivers); context (e.g., the salience of racial and ethnic issues in the community); and time (e.g., the 1990s versus the 1950s)" (p. 55). The focus on the proximal processes or what they call *activity settings* is particularly helpful because it zooms in on the circular and multi-determined interactions between the youth and their context to explore the fit between the context and the youth behavior. Zooming in on these activities allows for the identification of culture-related factors (e.g., *respeto, personalismo, humildad,* gender roles, and values) that impact specific interactions. The activity setting is the place in which adolescents must integrate, negotiate, and juggle all the different expectations of their peers, family, culture of origin, and host culture.

These authors have an interesting take on what we sometimes see in clinical practice, namely parents sending their children to live with extended family when the child is struggling. Children sometimes cite this decision as "proof" that they are not loved by their parents. Children may feel that the parents are just trying to get rid of them. The Koss and Vargas frame on this decision is that Latine parents are sometimes truly contextualists. Parents understand that a change in the contexts and in the specific set of activities the child is involved in daily (e.g., socializing with risk-taking peers) can be as powerful a determinant of the child's well-being as anything that is internal to the child (e.g., emotion regulation, anger, sadness). It is an important reminder of why the culturally competent therapist must *learn from the family* and their understanding of their unique circumstances before we use our traditional formulations to prematurely judge the family's actions.

Structural Family Therapy

An entire generation of systems thinkers such as Jay Haley, Nathan Ackerman, Carl Whitaker, Virginia Satir, Murray Bowen, Don Jackson, and Gregory Bateson made extraordinary contributions to the field of family therapy. Family theorists such as Monica McGoldrick, Marlene Watson, Kenneth Hardy, Celia Falicov, Paulette Hines, Nancy Boyd-Franklin, and so many others who put culture, race, and diversity front and center in the formulations about families have had an influence that cannot be overstated.

Structural Family Therapy (Minuchin & Fishman, 1981) brings many complex systems concepts to the front lines of practice and is a foundation of CIFFTA's family therapy work. Concepts such as circularity and complementarity are key to family work because they highlight how the behaviors of different family members fit together like a puzzle and serve to elicit, trigger, and reinforce each other. Because of circularity and complementarity, a therapist can often change one person's behavior by changing the other person's behavior first. For example, a person who habitually flees a disagreement may routinely trigger the partner to pursue vigorously in a desperate attempt to reach resolution. But the more one pursues, the more the other flees. The behavior of the pursuer can be modified by helping the other to avoid fleeing and to reach resolution more effectively. Given the concept of circularity, change can also come about by reducing the pursuit behavior first.

Theoretical contributions such as hierarchy and structure help the therapist to see how family relationship patterns shed light on who is in charge and who is following. It reminds us that parental figures should be in charge and leading/guiding and encourages the therapist to assess whether parental figures are doing this effectively. When children are shown to be more powerful in key interactions and therefore, higher on the power continuum/hierarchy, we know that this can lead to behavior problems. Understanding boundaries, the therapist can observe behavior and see how people intrude into areas that they shouldn't (e.g., kids violating the boundaries of the couple by getting involved in intimate partner issues).

Contributions such as alliances and coalitions help the therapist to see recurring patterns of support and attack that do not allow dyadic communication and resolution of disagreements, and that place key members at a disadvantage. Sometimes it becomes evident that a youngster enters a coalition with one parent against another and this can only hurt the youngster. The idea of proximity allows the therapist to be mindful that they can choose to work with the family in different ways depending on the need and situation. By shifting from a distant expert to interacting from a proximal position, the therapist can increase the intensity and power of their words. Joining, restructuring, and unbalancing all allow the therapist to think about how to enter and modify the interactions that are maintaining the problem or at least constraining the solutions that might otherwise emerge. This should whet the appetite of the reader who wants to read a gem in family therapy (*Family Therapy Techniques*, 1981) to better understand the underlying principles of Structural Family Therapy.

Family Research at the Spanish Family Guidance Center/ Center for Family Studies

The work on Brief Strategic Family Therapy (BSFT; Szapocznik & Kurtines, 1989; Santisteban et al., 2003, 2006) placed a therapy focused on Latine families on the map of evidence-based treatments. BSFT works to ensure that therapy fit with the family orientation of the Latine parents and worked to include all family members in therapy sessions. The work on engagement of family members who may be reluctant to enter treatment was one of the most significant breakthroughs in this work (Szapocznik et al., 1988). Beyond just stating that engagement of multiple family members was important, this work emphasized that the clinical work began not once a family was sitting in the therapy room but with the very first contact to schedule a session. The therapist was taught to begin the process of diagnosing family interactions and dynamics from the very first phone call. By learning to identify specific patterns of reluctance to engagement, the therapist can use specialized interventions for engagement that fit the family dynamics and circumstances (Santisteban & Szapocznik, 1994; Santisteban, 2008). As we described earlier in the case of motivation enhancement, the therapist must clearly identify and classify the pattern of reluctance (e.g., powerful adolescent, a caregiver preferring to keep out another caregiver) to know which specialized intervention to use. Research showed that the timely use of these specialized engagement strategies and techniques could significantly increase the number of families who entered and were retained in treatment (Coatsworth et al., 2001; Santisteban et al., 1996).

At a higher theoretical level, it is helpful to think about the fact that the family system has accepted the therapist into their system and *a new therapeutic system has formed* (Santisteban & Szapocznik, 1994). The formation of the therapeutic system begins the moment the family makes the initial phone call for an appointment, and it continues to develop as the therapist and family begin to meet. There can be many incompatibilities between the unique characteristics of certain families and the therapist's habitual ways of joining with clients. For example, a very relaxed therapist may realize that the very traditional family is not responding well to a less formal approach to engagement. By highlighting the therapist's role during the formation of the therapeutic system, what might otherwise be called *resistance, pathology,* or *lack of motivation* on the part of the client, requires a more complex analysis that includes the therapist's strategies and maneuvers to initiate therapy.

Some questions that you may ask yourself about the new therapeutic system might be:

1. "How does a family member's position within the family change because of having established a relationship with me?"
2. "How does my entry into the system dislodge key family members from their accustomed positions?"
3. "How can my position within this new system increase or decrease the chances each member will engage in and benefit from therapy?"
4. "Is any family member's role and power in the family threatened by my entry into the system?"
5. "How does each member want to use me to change the balance of power within the family?"
6. "How can my approach exacerbate or crystallize the fears and perceptions that are troubling this family?" (Santisteban & Szapocznik, 1994).

Multidimensional Ecosystemic Comparative Approach

Falicov (2017) provides a framework for formulating the meaning of migration, acculturation, religion, ecological context, and Latine family life cycles. The Multidimensional Ecosystemic Comparative Approach (MECA) takes a deep dive into the culture-related processes while always maintaining an ecological lens. Falicov reminds us that Latine immigrants don't always leave home behind as they move to a new country, and that many Latines juggle the two sets of cultures, values, and customs rather than replace one with another. MECA emphasizes the importance of *migration history* (including the age of migration and whether the family had segmented migration that separated family members in the process), *ecological context* (an appreciation of factors such as social class, race, occupation, education, social support and immigration status), *family organization* (including within family processes like blended families and parenting practices), and *family life cycle* (including transitions and the development of new roles within the family). All are essential perspectives that impact our work.

SUMMARY

In this chapter we presented what we believe to be key pillars in culturally informed work with Latine adolescents and families. In each section we attempted to show how different advances and contributions work their way into the treatment process and how therapists can use this knowledge to ensure competent and culturally informed work. Whether from an individual, family, or contextual perspective, we have highlighted the ways in which theorists, clinicians, and researchers have expanded on this work by integrating a cultural perspective that brings richness and ecological validity to the work.

The importance of connecting to the client's worldview and way of thinking about the problem and the solution cannot be overstated given how much our field values the development of a strong therapeutic alliance (Horvath & Greenberg, 1994). Some of the major components of therapeutic alliance are (1) client and therapist agreement on *Goals* of treatment, (2) client and therapist agreement on how to achieve the goals or *Task agreement,* and (3) the development of a personal *bond* between the therapist and client. Agreement on the nature of the underlying problem (especially when one is using a relational and contextual frame and not just the presenting problem) is an important step prior to deciding on the goals for treatment. A therapy process that facilitates eliciting of the client's perspective and preferences and uses it as a foundation for a collaborative process of treatment planning is likely to be one that has a real opportunity to build a strong therapeutic alliance. This is especially important with marginalized families who may not feel great about their treatment options, their past experiences with the therapy system, or feel coerced into treatment by systems such as the juvenile justice system.

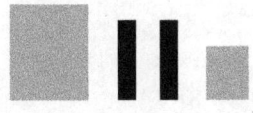

CIFFTA PRACTICE GUIDE

4

Preparing the Ground for CIFFTA Implementation

Before diving into each CIFFTA component that you will learn and add to your therapy toolbox (i.e., family therapy, individual therapy, and psychoeducational modules) it is helpful to cover issues that set the backdrop for successful CIFFTA implementation. This chapter will help you become more mindful of key abilities, skills, processes, and implementation decisions that make a difference. Whether a beginner or a seasoned therapist, it is important to stop and reflect on the factors that can facilitate or hinder treatment delivery.

UNIQUE ASPECTS OF FAMILY THERAPY

Because we work with therapists and programs that are not accustomed to implementing family therapy, we are often asked what is unique about family work. One of the most important aspects is preparing for the systemic forces that you will experience when doing family therapy. Entering a family system is a bit like going into the ocean for a swim. The swimmer can enter casually but may soon be surprised by the strength of the currents and how forcefully they move the swimmer around. The swimmer may only become aware of how far the currents have carried them when they come to shore to dry off and realize they have no idea where their towel is. When the swimmer makes the decision to swim into deep waters and far from the safety of the shore, it is particularly wise to have an accurate assessment of the currents and waves. This should be an informed decision based on how strong a swimmer they are and their capacity to get out of trouble.

As the therapist experiences the currents running through a family, they also appreciate how other family members are impacted. When things are not going well in families, family processes can feel like rip currents threatening to overpower individual family members trying to individuate and chart their own path. When things are going well, the family process can feel more like a lazy river allowing individuals to lie back and enjoy their travels through life. Most of the time individuals find themselves somewhere in between these two extremes, and they are often unaware of the power of these currents and their impact on their own well-being. It is the job of the therapist to identify when the currents are constraining progress and development and to consider how to harness the family currents so that they support the growth and well-being of all its members.

As is the case with the swimmer, therapists must honestly assess their own capacity to handle powerful family issues (e.g., coalitions, trauma, intense conflict) as they decide how deeply to delve into powerful family dynamics. The therapist should not begin to deliver services that are beyond their training and expertise. Opening painful wounds should only be done when you have the strategies and techniques to move negative interactions in a positive and healthy direction. In Chapter 6 you will learn the value of reframing, blocking, and reshaping enactments and how these tools allow you to maneuver in painful or highly conflictual interactions. Work in the most intense aspects of family therapy requires mastery of these strategies and techniques.

Doherty (1995) provides an instructive set of guidelines on how you can involve family members in educational interventions at lower levels of intensity and be mindful before delving into very intensive and conflict-laden interactions that require more expertise. CIFFTA provides the tools to address the most powerful family dynamics but merely reading a book does not replace the intensive training, coaching, and experience needed to prepare the therapist for what Doherty categorizes as Level 5 work. This level moves into couple and family of origin issues, and intense interpersonal conflicts with a mission of changing these relationships and interactions. Doherty shows how therapists can get into trouble if they go into more depth (Levels 4 and 5) than they are trained for and become overwhelmed and unable to exit competently. The family may also feel that they have been taken into deeper subjects than they had agreed to address.

DEVELOPING THE KNOWLEDGE, ABILITIES, AND SKILLS NEEDED TO IMPLEMENT CIFFTA

To date, CIFFTA therapists have been mostly master's-level trained family therapists, mental health counselors, clinical social workers, or PhD/PsyD-level psychologists. The seasoned family therapist can use this book and its tools to help families with many different issues. A therapist that is less experienced in working with complex family issues will need to acquire more intensive training and support. While approached to train bachelor's-level counselors who have a certification in the field of addiction, we believe these candidates need a higher level of training and more years of well-supervised experience working with youth and families if they are to be successful. The minimal initial training on an EBT is typically a 2- to 3-day in-person training event with an expert on the EBT or training on an online platform such as the one CIFFTA has available through Training and Implementation Associates (TIA). You can learn more about the CIFFTA online training platform by following this link: *www.guilford.com/santisteban-materials*. CIFFTA's state-of-the-art platform moves beyond knowledge acquisition, having the learner interact and practice interventions with simulated families, and receiving expert feedback (Chapter 9 provides more about this training resource).

While training is a major component of the adoption and implementation process, it is only the beginning of the process. It has been a mistake in the field to plan and allocate resources for training alone, as if *exposure* (Simpson, 2002) to a new treatment can lead to successful implementation and sustainment. Ongoing coaching and support are critically important so that a family therapist can reach the point where they can confidently use sophisticated strategies and interventions in complex and volatile clinical situations. Support often comes in the form of a strong supervisor, coaching and support from the model developers, and/or it may come in the form of a learning collaborative, consultation group, or peer learning network. We believe that one of the benefits of a lower-cost platform for the initial training phase is that it allows resources to be allocated to the complementary coaching and support phase. Furthermore, we strongly encourage that all therapists implementing the CIFFTA treatment be engaged with at least one of the supports mentioned above. In the sections that follow we describe therapist knowledge, abilities, and skills that are needed.

Developing a Systemic Perspective

When we are asked about the qualities of a good CIFFTA therapist, we usually start by stressing the importance of a strong systemic and relational perspective. This allows therapists to identify relational dynamics that impact behavior such as family systems, environmental and contextual stressors, discrimination, racism, and anti-immigrant messaging (e.g., Uri Bronfenbrenner and the Social Ecology Model). Using this perspective, the therapist learns to reduce risk factors while also mobilizing protective factors such as support from extended family, church families, and relationships that have been ruptured but can be repaired.

Our work to develop and fine-tune a family therapist's systemic perspective does not negate the reality that individuals have unique dispositions and personalities. Instead, it focuses on how the individual and contextual forces are constantly interacting to impact behavior. The contextual factors sometimes constrain options and sometimes exacerbate individual characteristics. One example that we often use is of an employee who is underperforming and seems depressed. There can be vulnerabilities to depression in the employee. But we will inevitably think differently about the problem if we find out that the boss is making unwanted sexual advances, that the employee has gone to human resources and has gotten no support, and that the employee was recently passed up for a promotion because they "made trouble." In helping this client, a systemic perspective opens more avenues for understanding the problem and for intervening. It is not a matter of deciding whether it is the contextual *or* the individual factor that must be changed, it becomes a matter of focusing on how the many factors interact around a particular situation. Figure 4.1 shows a Systemic Conceptualization Form that we use to document and keep present the many contextual forces that are impacting the youth, family, and their behavior.

Interestingly, less experienced therapists are often more open to learning and fully implementing a new systemic therapy. This may be because they enter without having competing and clashing habits, frameworks, and theoretical models. It may sometimes be stressful for therapists to try to implement a systemic, relational, and contextual therapy when that framework seems and feels inconsistent with an existing philosophical perspective. A therapist who is very strongly committed to an individually oriented approach may have a more difficult time prioritizing contextual factors and choosing to intervene at the systemic level.

Knowing Yourself as a Therapist

In preparing for complex family therapy, it is also helpful to attend to the person of the therapist, their history, and their personal characteristics (Bitter, 2014). Because therapists are the vehicle through which

CIFFTA Systemic Conceptualization Form

Presenting problems _____
_____

Adolescent
Underlying difficulties _____
_____

Strengths _____
_____

Family influences (parents, siblings, spouse, extended family)
Risk _____
_____

Protective _____
_____

Community/societal influences (school, neighborhood)
Risk _____
_____

Protective _____
_____

FIGURE 4.1. Conceptualizing treatment using contextual and systemic influences.

a treatment is delivered, therapists should become increasingly aware of themselves as people and identify strengths as well as possible blind spots that can impact family work. This is the reason many family therapy training programs require that students seek their own therapy as part of the program. For example, a therapist who may have grown up in a home with domestic violence, considerable substance use, or intense conflict, may not see similar situations clearly. They may have more difficulty responding therapeutically if they have unresolved issues in that specific area. The therapist must have addressed the issue well enough so that exposure to that specific topic in a new family does not trigger a reaction that interferes with effective therapy. Some reactions may be as subtle as avoiding disagreements and/or topics that should be allowed to emerge in the family. The dynamics of a family are powerful, and it is easy to miss how the therapist is drawn into the *rip currents* of the family.

Likewise, a therapist must be very aware of whether they tend to favor one or another side in a family system. For example, some therapists may tend to ally with younger family members more easily than with parental figures or vice versa. This type of preference can make it more difficult to effectively handle the multiple alliances that a family therapist must juggle. Success at juggling multiple alliances without losing family members is one of the hallmarks of a good family therapist. This competence sets family therapy apart from individual therapy. Support for one side or another in family work must only occur if it is done strategically to help move the family system toward more flexibility and should not occur because the therapist feels more comfortable with certain family members.

Developing Comfort with Being Directive

In systemic family therapies such as CIFFTA, it is important for the therapist to feel comfortable with being directive. It does not mean that the therapist should be central to all interactions in the room. In fact, we often want the therapist to sit back, become less central, and let the family do the work that changes family interactions under the direction of the therapist. However, the therapist must have the capacity to jump into the interactions to reshape and redirect the conversations and communications *in vivo*. One of the biggest mistakes a family therapist can make is to sit back for too long while negativity and hostility is expressed with few guardrails. If vulnerable family members are hurt in these interactions and the therapist is passive, it is easy to imagine that shame and hopelessness increase, and family members will refuse to return. One of Minuchin's (1981) outstanding contributions touches on the way a therapist must be flexible and capable in the use of distance and proximity in the therapy room. Minuchin argued for the importance of a therapist taking different positions in the family system, including close or proximal positions, median positions, and more distant/expert positions. It is not that the therapist chooses which position feels best for them in general, it is that the therapist practices how to move from one position to another even when some positions are out of their comfort zone. *The more the position is determined by the needs of the family and the therapy process, and less by the needs and idiosyncrasies of the therapist, the more effective the therapist will be.*

GROUNDWORK NEEDED TO PREPARE FOR CIFFTA IMPLEMENTATION

CIFFTA has been tested and implemented in several different ways including as an early intervention for behavior problems (Santisteban et al., 2017, 2022; Mena et al., 2023), as a treatment for self-harm behavior (Mena et al., 2024a; Santisteban et al., 2024), and as a treatment for substance use and co-occurring disorders (Santisteban et al., 2011). The empirically supported engagement strategies published by Daniel A. Santisteban and colleagues are also key to CIFFTA implementation (Coatsworth et al., 2001; Santisteban et al., 1994, 1996). CIFFTA's format and intensity change depending on the presenting problems and the severity of the adolescent and family risk factors. Table 4.1 shows the differences in treatment format. CIFFTA consists of three different components and two important guidelines are to maintain the momentum of therapy (e.g., not missing weeks of therapy that disrupts the momentum of change) and that no component be neglected. Fewer total sessions should not mean that a specific component is left out. The balance of components is integral and should always be maintained unless there is a clinical reason for adjusting the number of individual sessions with the youth (e.g., work with a younger child may lead to more family sessions while a youth with very low motivation to change may need additional individual sessions).

A recent real-world implementation of the CIFFTA Family Strengthening Program (Mena et al., 2024b) showed the flexibility of the program. The program team treated a wide range of presenting problems, and the treatment was delivered by experienced master's-level family therapists over a 12- to 16-week period. The length of treatment and number of sessions varied depending on the risk level of the adolescent and the family (see Table 4.1). *Families were considered at high risk*

TABLE 4.1. CIFFTA Length and Frequency of Treatment

Adolescents with less severe symptoms	Adolescents with more severe symptoms
4–6 sessions per month	8 sessions per month (2 per week)
3- to 4-month period (14–23 sessions)	4-month period (24–32 sessions)
60-minute sessions	60-minute sessions

when lower levels of family cohesion, higher levels of family conflict, suicidal ideation, suicide attempts, self-harm, risky sexual behavior and/or substance use, and higher level of adolescent behavior problems were reported. Their optimal and recommended intensity was two sessions every week for 4 months of treatment. *Families were considered at lower risk* when presenting with lower levels of family conflict and higher levels of family cohesion and reporting lower levels of adolescent behavior problems. For low-risk cases, therapists were expected to deliver three sessions every 2 weeks (i.e., one family session weekly and either an individual or psychoeducation session every other week).

Within CIFFTA, family therapy sessions are the most delivered intervention, typically occurring every week. Individual therapy sessions with the Adolescent and Psychoeducational module sessions are typically staggered. Module delivery may focus on different family subsystems (e.g., caregivers only, adolescent only, or all family members) and are selected depending on the family's unique clinical and cultural circumstances. Invariably we find that therapists have their preferences for certain modules and for certain components of the model (e.g., family, individual, or psychoeducation). However, the power of CIFFTA is based on using all three components so that they create synergy and reinforce each other, and that module selection be based on the unique needs and preferences of the family and not the therapist. Monitoring of implementation keeps a careful watch on this balance and process. For example, ensuring that sufficient family therapy sessions are implemented may be most important when services are delivered in a school system in which it is easier to offer services only during the day or in an agency that does not have evening hours. This is also the case when therapists are first learning family therapy and may shy away from complex engagement issues. These patterns of service delivery constrain the use of family therapy that should include caregivers who are working, and special preparation is needed to ensure the family receives those services that would be most beneficial. Ensuring that staff are willing and able to work after hours is key. If these aspects are not monitored and addressed, it is easy for implementation to include very few family therapy sessions.

Using the Modular Approach and Tailoring Profile Effectively

CIFFTA requires that the therapist/agency identify the unique client characteristics that can lead to tailoring treatment. A key to our work is the Tailoring Profile that identifies key issues (e.g., depression, substance use, self-harm, and immigration-related separations) and client characteristics (e.g., LGBTQ+ youth, blended families, and acculturation profile) that should inform treatment planning. This information guides the use of CIFFTA components, including psychoeducational modules that address the themes that are highlighted as important to each youth and family. A *shared decision-making process* ensures that the family's input and preferences are an essential part of the tailoring process. This type of collaborative process can go a long way toward generating family buy-in, engagement, and a strong therapeutic alliance. The therapist can say, "Based on the things you and your family have shared with me and with our assessment team, I believe that you may find these three modules helpful. I would like to know whether you want to hear more about how this material might help with the situations you described. You might even help me rank the modules in terms of relevance and priorities." Ensuring that client preferences and perspectives are systematically considered encourages the family and therapist to agree on what the problem is, what the treatment should include, and what the outcome of treatment should be.

The steps that support the tailoring process include (1) using self-report or interviews that can identify information to facilitate treatment planning and tailoring, (2) creating a client-tailoring profile that links client information to treatment goals and a treatment plan, and (3) utilizing different CIFFTA treatment components and modules to carry out the treatment plan. It helps to have a solid fit between the tailoring variables and the treatment options available within the model. It does not help very much to identify a complex problem (e.g., acculturation conflict or racism) and then not offer the therapist a tool that can help to address that problem with the youth and the family. This approach also reminds us that when using a *culturally centered or culturally adapted* treatment, the therapist can easily err by using a "one-size-fits-all-Latines" approach. Even characteristics that are prominent among Latines (e.g., familism, collectivism, religiosity, and *respeto*) are not endorsed by every family. Familism, traditionalism, and religiosity may be endorsed by many Latine families, but this does not mean that it is endorsed by the unique family sitting in your treatment room. In the room you must remain humble and curious to detect the specifics of the family's values, beliefs, and behaviors that should be considered in treatment.

The CIFFTA Tailoring Report (see Figure 4.2) provides the clinician with relevant information about the adolescents and their families, information based on the family's reports at intake and on the CIFFTA Clinical Interview (described later in the chapter). The report flags areas of concern that can be addressed, protective factors that can be enhanced, and unique family conditions that should be considered in treatment.

Adolescent demographics	
Age	15
Gender	Female/cisgender
Sexual orientation	Heterosexual/straight
Family	
Parent–child separations	Yes—4 years
Marital/couple separation	Yes
Parenting	Poor
Parental stress	Yes
Parental communication	Good
Parental involvement	Good
Adolescent functioning	
Conduct problems	No
Depression	Yes
Anxiety	Yes
Substance use	No
Emotion regulation	Poor
Traumatic experiences	No
School functioning	Poor
Peer relationships	Poor
Environmental stressors	
Acculturation stress	Yes
Immigration stress	No
Discrimination	No
Motivation for treatment/change	
	Good

FIGURE 4.2. Example of a CIFFTA Tailoring Report.

The Tailoring Report provides the therapist a summary of such areas as:

- Adolescent emotional and behavioral issues, substance use, and self-harm
- Adolescent problem recognition and motivation to change
- Family functioning
- Environmental stressors such as occupational stress, marital stress, discrimination stress, and immigration stress

- Family composition: single parent, blended family
- School problems: suspensions, bullying, and academic failure
- Trauma: Presence of traumatic events

Areas that are elevated on CIFFTA's Tailoring Report can be addressed using its psychoeducational modules. The module options allow you to respond to the tailoring report with a customized treatment that addresses the unique issues presented by your client. For example, if only depression, self-harm, and acculturation conflicts are present, the family's treatment plan should focus on the corresponding modules. In many Latine families the acculturation gap scale score is high on the HSI (Cervantes et al., 2011), meaning that there is a discrepancy in the Latine values, beliefs, and customs endorsed by caregivers and the youth. To address this, the CIFFTA therapist recommends use of the Acculturation module. This module provides a way of explaining how acculturation differences can impact family relationships (i.e., arguments, disconnection, language barriers) and serves to normalize the acculturation-related tensions being experienced by the family. When caregivers understand that youth are showing a *normal* and frequently occurring pattern of acculturation, they take the changes less personally and not as a rejection of their values and culture. Later in family therapy sessions, the family can work through the impact of acculturation on their specific family with less intensity. By successfully addressing the acculturation issue, you are removing a problem that is further complicating the effectiveness of parenting and that is creating enough stress that it impacts a youth's presenting complaints, such as depression and self-harm. Having received modules on Acculturation, Depression, Self-Harm, and a Parenting module, the family has increased readiness to address the current circumstances in a more adaptive way.

The only module that we tend to give to all families, regardless of the profile, is the Parenting module (for caregivers only). We believe that all caregivers should receive this module early in treatment, immediately after the engagement and joining phase. The Parenting module emphasizes areas that are central to healthy family functioning, caregiver–youth relationships, adolescent development, parental supervision and monitoring, appropriate rewards and consequences, healthy communication, and how to validate the youth. The work of caregivers in a family with a youth seeking treatment is complex enough that we feel the Parenting module is always a basic piece of the treatment puzzle. The content received by caregivers sets the stage for later family sessions as well as for all other modules.

The tailoring profile and modular component support CIFFTA's *transdiagnostic* approach. This means that the therapy can work to address a variety of problems and that you do not need to have a different therapy for each specific presenting complaint, such as depression, substance use, or self-harm. CIFFTA modules address different types of presenting problems using the same framework. Treatment targets the same "maintaining mechanisms" (e.g., family maladaptive relationship patterns, invalidation, high conflict, emotion dysregulation, low motivation to change) that may underlie several co-occurring disorders. By utilizing psychoeducational modules that are consistent with the needs of the youth and families, addressing maintaining mechanisms that can constrain change, and by using a joint decision-making process in the selection of treatment targets, the unique presenting symptoms can be fully addressed.

In summary, a therapy process that facilitates eliciting of the client's perspective and preferences and uses it as a foundation for a collaborative process of treatment planning is likely to be one that has a real opportunity to build a strong therapeutic alliance and to positively impact outcomes. The profile guides the decision-making process on the best way to use the CIFFTA components, primarily the psychoeducational modules, but the counselor retains final choice in the selection in collaboration with the family. A collaborative approach is especially important with a population of Latine families (and other marginalized families) who are often not feeling great about their treatment options or their past experiences with the mental health system.

Creating Synergy among CIFFTA Treatment Components

A strength of the CIFFTA model is its ability to create synergy among the treatment components and to address the presenting and underlying problems from multiple angles to optimize outcomes. Here we discuss the creation of synergy as treatment addresses three types of presenting problems.

Adolescent with Substance Misuse

CIFFTA has been used effectively with adolescents who were referred to treatment by schools and/or the juvenile justice system because of substance misuse (Santisteban et al., 2011). In working with substance using youth, we often ran across a profile in which the youth and family endorse *high substance use risk, low problem recognition, and risky sexual behaviors*. In these cases, the CIFFTA treatment plan prioritizes individual sessions using MI to fully engage the adolescent and to work on increasing their recognition of the problem, increasing intrinsic motivation to change, and to select a target(s) for change before moving onto modules that tackle the risks of substance misuse and risky sexual behavior. As motivation to change increases, the therapist can proceed to describe to the client what the Substance Use and Risky Sex modules can offer, and clients can have a say about the direction they want to take in the next phase of their treatment.

We often find that neither the youth nor the caregivers have accurate and complete information about the characteristics and harmful effects of the substances being used or their possible consequences. Our Substance Use module offers the adolescent and separately the caregivers, information on the signs of use, on the effects of specific substances, and on the specific patterns of use. The module provides the information and vocabulary that can help caregivers better communicate with, lead, and guide their youngsters. It is often best to administer the modules separately because the youth often fail to ask questions or give facts about the pattern or context of use in front of the caregivers. This is particularly true early in the treatment process. On the other side, caregivers are sometimes reticent to admit how little they know about specific substances and their effect in front of the youth. Also, if the information is processed together early in treatment, caregivers sometimes blow up in a way that effectively shuts down the conversation with the youth before they disclose key facts about their use and the specific peers they use with. You can use the substance use module to provide both caregivers and youth the types of information that will facilitate more productive discussions in subsequent family and individual therapy sessions.

The work done in the psychoeducational sessions, which includes a Parenting module, is continued in individual and family sessions. In individual therapy sessions with the adolescent, you use MI to elicit and evoke the adolescent's own motivation to modify their patterns of use and to produce their own reasons why change might be necessary. It is the context in which the adolescent's ambivalence can emerge and be assessed calmly, without caregivers becoming frustrated. Substance use flags in the Tailoring Report typically mean that family therapy sessions must follow up on the generalization of the Parenting module skills and address how caregivers set rules for, monitor, and establish consequences for the youth. The work also identifies the parenting skills that work and do not work well in the family, how to improve communication around risky behavior so that it is open, honest, and not attacking, and handling the emergence of conflict and hostility in the family that erode trust. Effective leadership around substance use is key and the knowledge gained in the parenting and substance use psychoeducational sessions helps create the foundation for effective leadership. The re-establishment of honest communication and trust also become keys to treatment.

Adolescent Self-Harm

When working with youth reporting suicide ideation, attempts and other self-harm behaviors such as cutting, the therapist can use the Self-Harm module to ensure a full and accurate understanding of the different types of self-harm, intrapersonal and interpersonal contributing factors to self-harm and triggers, address the fear and stigma that might keep the problem hidden, and discuss ways that therapy can help using individual (e.g., emotion modulation/regulation, distress tolerance) and family (e.g., support, validation, and parenting skills) interventions. The Self-Harm module can be delivered to the youth and caregivers together or separately.

After the module, family therapy sessions will often need to focus on increased communication, validation, support, and instilling confidence that talking about urges to self-harm does not increase risk. It must also reduce the sense of desperation, helplessness, and hopelessness that emerges in family members. You can use family therapy sessions to shape family interactions into more validating, adaptive, and supportive relationships. By providing the psychoeducational information prior to focusing on these issues in family and individual sessions, family members are more open and ready to process the self-harm and to work on alternate ways to manage the triggers to self-harm. Also, as you create an environment in which communication becomes less hostile and intense, you will see how adolescents become more willing to admit to certain self-harm urges, triggers, and behaviors.

Immigration-Related Separations

If we identify that this same youth was separated for an extended period of time from a primary caregiver during the process of immigration and has never been the same, that immigration experience is not a tangential "layer" outside of the core issue of treatment. The client's experience should be a major focus of the treatment because it can directly impact family relationships, despair, and hopelessness. In fact, what we have learned is that if a therapist skips the topic of the separation and begins to work on other areas of concern (i.e., self-harm and family conflict), little progress is made, and the family becomes frustrated and loses hope. Conversely, if the therapist begins with the Separations module and then progresses to family sessions that allow family members to communicate their experiences together, we see improved treatment progress. The remaining work related to increasing motivation, self-harm, improving family communication and connection is made that much easier.

Collecting Information That Facilitates the Tailoring Processes

The ability to tailor the treatment to the unique needs and preferences of the adolescent and families requires that applicable information be collected. It may not always be possible to collect all the information we mention below, but it is important to appreciate the potential value of each piece of information and use that to make informed decisions in designing your formal assessment of the client and family. There are valid, reliable, and easily accessible screening instruments and questionnaires for each of the areas. As we will show, the CIFFTA Clinical Interview is a way of filling in gaps and collecting a limited amount of data in important areas that we were unable to assess in depth by other means. The key is to know what questions to ask and what data to seek so that you can identify *the clinical and cultural factors that make a treatment process and outcome difference* and that should be used in tailoring the treatment plan.

Adolescent Presenting Problem Data

A first step is to correctly assess the clinical symptoms that are part of the youth's presenting complaint(s). Some family therapists will argue against placing emphasis on an individual's clinical presentation or diagnosis because it detracts from the systemic focus on family interactions that may elicit and maintain the behaviors. We believe that the therapist can balance a focus on the individual and the system. Substance misuse, depression, anxiety, self-harm behavior, and behavior problems such as conduct disorder are issues you will frequently encounter. For example, you can screen for depression and anxiety using the Patient Health Questionnaire–9 (PHQ-9; Richardson et al., 2010) and the Generalized Anxiety Disorder–7 (GAD-7; Casares et al., 2024). These screening tools are available for free and can be downloaded from their respective websites. Whenever possible, use valid diagnostic and clinical screening and assessment tools and procedures (Cervantes & Bui, 2015) and select measures that include youth and caregiver reports on the same behaviors. It is helpful to obtain information from multiple perspectives. Although space limitations hinder us from going more in depth into this issue, we should note that Geisinger (2015) and others have argued for the development of standardized psychological assessment measures developed specifically for Latines that go beyond translations of clinical assessment tools for assessing conditions such as anxiety and depression by incorporating an assessment of acculturation, cultural stress, and cultural beliefs about illness and recovery.

Adolescent Developmental Stage and Circumstances

Children and adolescents go through many changes due to their developmental stage and you will want to seek information on challenges and events that emerge frequently during the adolescent developmental stage. For example, youth are forming an identity across many fronts (e.g., ethnic, racial, sexual orientation, gender identity) and youth may fear that therapists are not comfortable with these conversations and/or will not be affirming and accepting. You will want to ask about sexually risky behavior and experimentation with substance use because experimentation occurs fairly frequently during adolescents and there may be a great deal of peer pressure (peers being an emerging and powerful influence) to experiment in ways that the youth is not fully comfortable with or thoughtful about. Substance use could be assessed using instruments such as the Timeline Followback interview (Robinson et al., 2014) or the CRAFFT (Car, Relax, Alone, Forget, Friends, Trouble; Bagley et al., 2017; Oesterle et al., 2015) screening tool. These screening tools are also available for free and can be downloaded from their respective websites. School-related and academic difficulties must be part of the assessment. Note that each of these assessments can lead to specific interventions that help the youth along in the developmental challenges and that help caregivers focus their support and guidance.

Assessing Motivation to Change

Adolescents sometimes seek treatment of their own accord, but it is often the case that they do not come in as a voluntary *and motivated client*. Often the initial client may be the concerned caregiver(s) who knows that things are not going well. Sometimes it is the school or juvenile justice system that may require that a youngster receive services due to a significant event that placed the youth in trouble with a system. You may work with diversion programs that offer treatment as an alternative to a legal consequence. Keep in mind that if a youth comes to see you as part of an agreement with the juvenile justice system, you may be perceived as part of the system that is *punishing* them for the transgression. It is key that you work through this initial perception and differentiate yourself from the referring system to increase the likelihood of a strong alliance and successful outcome. The important thing you must remember is that treatment progression and change will be hindered if the adolescent's motivation to rethink their behavior is low and if a power struggle ensues because you, the family, or an outside system are the only ones that think change is needed. Assessment of a youngster's motivation to change and an assessment of their stage of change should be an important part of your work.

Assessment of Family Relationship, History, and Family Life Cycle Stage

There are important family areas that you may want to assess. The work starts with having a good sense of who is considered *family* and getting a good sense of the quality of the relationships. Family therapists often recommend the use of a genogram (McGoldrick et al., 1999) although that can be a very intensive intervention of its own. Interestingly there are online applications for completing genograms that can save time, but the therapist must note that this information can be quite delicate, and its collection must be done with great clinical sensitivity. This is particularly true in Black and Latine families in which important relationships may be kin and not always formal or blood relationships (Boyd-Franklin, 2003). Furthermore, because blended families are so common in our society and come with such unique relationship implications, this is also an important area to explore. Blended families mean that certain dyads have more history together than others, and certain behaviors such as parenting and giving of affection may be easier with some family members than with others. This is an underappreciated set of dynamics in family work.

You will want to have a good handle on family structures and dynamics, including separated or divorced caregivers, and single-parent families. Youth can be stressed by loyalty requirements, and there may also be tensions between biological parents and/or other caregivers such as grandparents. Rather than seeing this as an insurmountable deficit, we view it as a clear opportunity to normalize any stress due to complex negotiations around caregiving, to improve the communication, cooperation, and support between caregivers, and to deepen the relationship by focusing on shared hopes and dreams for the youth's future, success, and well-being.

Assessment and appreciation of the family life cycle stage is important as each stage requires different abilities and sensitivities from the family members. A man who is a good partner is not necessarily prepared to be a good father when the child arrives. The role is something that may be quite different from anything that has been done before. Just as one cannot automatically expect that a good basketball player will be a good soccer or football player, one should not expect that a family member will be good in an entirely new role. The stress and conflict that can emerge is material for the family therapist. The same is true as the family moves to become a family with an adolescent, a family with a person with a disability or a major medical illness, and later an empty nest family in which the children have left, and the remaining family members must adjust to the new life circumstances. Often, families also need help when a family member is gone for an extended period and managing the re-entry of the family member can require substantial work. Such situations are encountered when a caregiver has been away as part of the military and when working with the children of inmates/prisoners. Having a full appreciation of the challenges that come with each stage, with the transition from one stage to another, and with reintegration is key to being a competent family therapist.

Acculturation Data

We have made the argument that cultural values, practices, and beliefs should be front and center when working with Latine clients. For this reason, therapists should consider the use of an acculturation measure so that the therapist can know the profile of the adolescent and the caregivers in terms of their endorsement of activities and values that represent either the host culture, the culture of origin, or both. These measures help us to understand not only individual acculturation profiles but also differences in the profiles within the family. Differences in acculturation between family members can contribute to relational and communication difficulties in the family. As we discussed in Chapter 2, it is important to select bidimensional measures that do not assume that host culture behaviors and values are necessarily *replaced* by the new host culture values and behaviors, but that also permit the individual to report being bicultural.

Immigration and Acculturation Stress Data

Although acculturation and acculturation stress are often used interchangeably, it is important to distinguish the two. Acculturation measures document an individual's endorsement of a society's values, behaviors, and beliefs. Stress measures related to immigration or acculturation measure the amount and type of stress that result from the process of immigration and acculturation.

CIFFTA's work has benefited from using the Hispanic Stress Inventory for adults and for youngsters (described in Chapter 2). The measures help to document the types of ecological and contextual stressors that adult and youth family members may be experiencing due to factors including immigration stress, acculturation stress, stress related to within-family differences on acculturation, economic stress, discrimination stress, parenting stress, and marital stress. Marital stress is a variable that becomes quite important when there are issues with parenting because it becomes particularly difficult to be on the same page parenting a youth when there is conflict in the couple that may be undermining the needed teamwork.

Although developed to a much lesser degree, we have also tried to measure protective factors and resilience in Latine families. In our recent work, we have moved to link contextual stressors to reported specific, contextual resilience strategies mentioned by Latine families in confronting acculturation stressors. We emphasize the importance of further *mobilizing* family strengths and traditional values into early intervention and prevention programs that can buffer the impact of weakening connection to traditional family protective factors (Castro et al., 2004).

The Role of the CIFFTA Clinical Interview

To facilitate the collection and incorporation of culture-related individual and family material, we developed the CIFFTA Clinical Interview. This interview can either complement the intake measures already collected by a therapist or agency or can substitute for such measures when the data could not be collected. The comprehensive semistructured interview is completed by the therapist in the early engagement sessions. A key to succeeding with the interview is to implement it in an engaging manner. It should be used to get to know the family and its history in a deep and respectful way. As with any data collection, if it is done in a robotic and bureaucratic fashion, it will be less effective and may even create distance from the family. The interview should be presented as a way of getting to know the family (i.e., engagement) and to identify the best ways that CIFFTA (and its psychoeducational modules) can be helpful to them. This history does not include a focus on intrapersonal dynamics that are related to the family, but instead family events that have had a direct impact on its members. The interview facilitates the sharing of information about family history, history of adolescent problems, and major cultural factors that have impacted the family.

The types of information that our interview focuses on include:

- The history of the family unit, where the parent-figures were born, when they formed as a couple, when the child(ren) were born, adopted, or brought into the family informally, any separations or divorces, separations between the children and caregivers, and couple conflict issues.
- The family's weekly routines (i.e., visits to extended family and or divorced parents) and if divorced, a description of what the routine looks like, and whether the caregivers share responsibilities for parenting.
- A sense of the closeness or distance in relationships. Who is closest to and supported by whom, who is distant from whom, who is in conflict/support with whom?

- Who takes on what parenting and caregiver roles (e.g., nurturing role and disciplinarian)? Has it always been like that, or has it changed? If there are multiple caregivers, how much do they agree on how to do it and how well do they work together?
- When did the child's problems emerge? What parenting interventions and strategies worked or did not work? What rules, chores, consequences, and rewards were present?

For immigrant families, there is a full immigration/acculturation and migration history to understand.

- Why did the family leave their country of origin (i.e., reasons, expectations)? What was life like back home (stress, violence, politics)? How did they arrive (route and dangers)? Who did they come with? Why and how was that decision made? What type of support was available upon arrival? What problems were encountered? Did they come together or were there separations due to immigration?
- How have the caregivers and family changed over time (values and behaviors)? Have there been different rates of adjustment/acculturation? Has that different profile of adjustment resulted in stress?
- What negatively perceived changes in the family's social and economic status have occurred? What are the stresses that resulted from related losses? Have there been any immigration/documentation problems? Were there changes in social networks?
- Is there currently a support system? Did/does the family perceive a sense of alienation, isolation, and/or discrimination? Are they connected with agencies that can be helpful with their documentation process? It is helpful for the therapist/agency to create a list of services available in the community around issues of immigration and documentation.
- What types of traumatic experiences have been experienced?

We should mention here that some of these questions, designed to help engage and get to know the family, can be threatening when the family feels vulnerable regarding documentation status and deportation. Only in a context of trust and knowing how the information will be stored and used will a family feel comfortable revealing such information. As a therapist, you must be very sensitive to instances where you should refrain from this level of inquiry so that the family is not pushed away. Using the information you collect, you can develop a preliminary tailored treatment plan. Then you can select, from all the CIFFTA components, strategies, and tools at your disposal, those that are most relevant for the youth and family that you are working with in treatment. Table 4.2 summarizes key goals of therapy and presents them by phase of treatment. The sequence is not set in stone or rigorously prescribed but are guidelines that should help you think about the therapy process.

TREATMENT IMPLEMENTATION AND DELIVERY DECISIONS

Traditional work with youth and families involves in-person and office-based services and this is the way CIFFTA was originally designed. There are benefits to office work, including increased control over the environment and potential distractions. In Chapter 6, we present the specialized engagement work (Santisteban et al., 1994, 1996) used by CIFFTA to engage reluctant family members and clients who may feel unwelcome or coerced into treatment. Suffice it to say that if the therapist is effective at conveying the importance and power of having family members attend office sessions to work on a specific problem, families are incredibly resourceful in getting to the office. The benefit to the family is that being in the office allows the therapist to use the full power of the treatment setting for the benefit of the client. This assumes that the therapist and office have flexible hours and have removed all other obvious obstacles to service utilization (e.g., limited hours of service, long waiting lists, and lack of space for family sessions).

Yet there are service delivery obstacles that have led the field to consider other options such as virtual delivery of the intervention and home-based therapy. This interest has been fueled by the natural desire to increase accessibility for clients who tend to underutilize services. In making these important decisions, therapists and agency leaders must weigh the pros and cons of each approach and the factors that impact both efficacy and safety. Here we will cover some of the practice issues to consider in virtual work and home-based work although we do not discuss legal or regulatory issues that vary by state.

Virtual Delivery of CIFFTA

Technology can augment treatments by addressing intervention delivery challenges (e.g., logistical challenges related to entire families getting to an office after hours for sessions), providing variable information formats (e.g., multimedia) that are engaging, reducing stigma related to office visits (Bischoff et al., 2004), and encouraging therapeutic work outside of formal session times (e.g., competing diary cards online and watching psychoeducational videos). CIFFTA was used and tested in a

TABLE 4.2. CIFFTA at a Glance

	Adolescent modules and individual therapy	Family modules and family therapy
Engagement and joining (pretreatment and sessions 1–2)	• Validating reluctance to participate • Specialized engagement strategies • Increasing collaborative work to cocreate the therapy • Build trust and instill hope	• Systemic conceptualization of the problem • Validating reluctance to participate • Engagement strategies • Increasing collaborative work to cocreate the therapy • Build trust and instill hope
Increasing motivation to change (sessions 1–3)	• Stages-of-change evaluation—Motivation to change • Motivational enhancement	• Stages-of-change evaluation—motivation to change • Motivational enhancement
Knowledge sharing/health information modules (sessions 3–5)	• Behavioral and mental health symptoms (e.g., depression, anxiety, ADHD, substance use, self-harm) • Effects of acculturation, family member separations • Ethnic/racial identity and societal acceptance/rejection • Understanding social media, legal and school systems	• Behavioral and mental health symptoms (e.g., depression, anxiety, ADHD, substance use, self-harm) • Effects of acculturation, family member separations • Ethnic/racial identity and societal acceptance/rejection • Understanding social media, legal and school systems
Decrease negative and conflictual family interactions (sessions 3–24)	• Decreased hostility and aggression • Improve conflict resolution skills • Identify triggers to anger and conflictual interactions	• Decreased hostility and aggression by shaping family interactions • Improved conflict resolution • Identify triggers to anger and conflictual interactions
Increase supportive family interactions (sessions 3–24)	• More openness to parental influence • Validating communication • Expressing care and support	• Understanding youth vulnerabilities and stressors • Shaping interactions to include validation communication, and expression of care, support, protection
Skills development modules (sessions 5–24)	• Interpersonal effectiveness • Emotion regulation • Goal setting • Distress tolerance	• Parenting • Communication • Guidance, leadership, and monitoring
Maintenance and relapse prevention (sessions 13–24)	• Monitoring triggers to anger and to conflictual family relationships • Trusting new skills that have been mastered	• Monitoring triggers to conflictual family relationships • Trusting new skills that have been mastered

hybrid delivery with technology used to deliver the psychoeducational modules (Santisteban et al., 2017). At the time we did not recommend fully virtual delivery of the treatment.

When COVID-19 emerged and in-person sessions were not feasible, our team developed guidelines for the use of technology to deliver all therapy sessions (Mena et al., 2024a). One key issue that emerged is the need to ensure safety in virtual treatment sessions. It is helpful to develop an emergency plan with each family at the start of treatment that includes dialing 911 if the clinician feels that the youth or caregiver are in danger to themselves or others. When working with an adolescent in a telehealth session, we strongly recommend that a caregiver be present in the home and/or that the therapist have the caregiver contact information.

Virtual sessions must also deal with challenges that are present in home-based work including having specific strategies for providing structure for the sessions and for handling distractions (e.g., dogs, neighbors, TV, cooking) that can derail the therapy sessions. Sometimes distractions just happen (e.g., a neighbor knocking on the door or a peer visiting) and sometimes the clients use the distractions to reduce the intensity of the session and as a way of avoiding certain issues. Structuring the sessions can include ways to ensure privacy when that is needed. You should plan the use of space so that individual sessions with the adolescent can enjoy privacy. You can do a great deal of work upfront including discussing the telehealth setup, assessing connectivity, and privacy with all members.

The fully virtual delivery of family sessions is even more difficult than the delivery of individual and psychoeducational sessions. You must plan for there to be enough space for a family session in which several individuals can be in front of the camera. Watching for family interaction patterns is a bit more challenging. As in any telehealth environment, it is important to be keenly aware of nonverbal cues and facial expressions. It is often necessary for the therapist to move close to the camera, to convey that the therapist is engaged and empathizing.

The use of the Zoom "share screen" tool and the whiteboard features are particularly helpful with adolescents. Any type of "annotation" feature, such as can be found on Zoom, can keep the clients engaged. This type of interactive process is particularly needed because the psychoeducation sessions are didactic in nature. The therapist cannot risk losing the client because they passively sit and listen to a face on a screen. Constant checking in with the client and use of the discussion questions also help keep the client's attention. When using an online platform for therapy sessions, it is important to ensure that it is HIPAA compliant to protect confidentiality. Lastly, it is imperative to objectively assess early on whether each component (family, individual, and psychoeducation) of the CIFFTA treatment can be delivered effectively virtually and, if not, a conversation with the family must occur to determine how best to proceed with treatment.

Home-Based Family Therapy

Many programs have moved to home-based service delivery as a way of reaching families who are physically unable to travel to the office and families who cannot take the time to travel. Some therapists feel that visiting the home gives them much more information that can be used in assessing safety and in treatment planning. Visiting the home can also help them better understand the family and the family's circumstances. Indeed, a therapist who suggests that certain therapy tasks be completed in the home can benefit from having a more complete understanding of the conditions of the home (e.g., limited space, insufficient quiet spaces, and lack of privacy). Finally, some therapists feel that families receiving in-home services have a stronger sense that the therapist really cares about them.

The decision to conduct home-based work should not be made without a full consideration of the factors that may negatively impact the therapeutic process and therapeutic outcomes. As Christensen (1995) pointed out, therapist concerns about obstacles inherent in home-based work are not always considered in the equation. Among the obstacles were distractions in the home that impeded or slowed the changes sought and concerns that therapist's safety could negatively impact the work because there was less confrontation of sensitive issues in the client's home. Some therapists reported trying to finish the work with the family by early afternoon (e.g., 2:30 P.M.), but it is difficult to expect all family members to be present at that time. Others have also reported issues with therapist feelings of safety and comfort and the risk that this can negatively impact self-reported level of therapeutic alliance (Glebova et al., 2012). One should consider whether a therapist distracted and stressed by the travel from one home to another and safety issues might also be less attentive to the complex processes at work in families and therapy. Getting to the location and dealing with other concerns requires so much energy that little is left for the actual therapy work.

We believe that often teams move too quickly to home-based work based on the assumption it is always better for families and because they run into difficulties engaging reluctant family members. Too often there is a knee-jerk reaction that office-based work is only about therapist comfort and ignores the needs of the family. We must acknowledge that the decision to leave the office comes at a price. Sessions in the office tend to have fewer distractions and therapists have more control over the factors that can lead to positive family changes in perspective and behaviors. The power of the therapist to bring about a new experience may be greater in the office. Furthermore, the time and resources required to have a therapist drive around large cities often means that fewer families can be served, and that the therapist's attention can suffer. All these factors should be considered in making an informed decision regarding service delivery.

One Therapist or Several?

One of the consequential decisions is whether to have the same therapist deliver both individual and family therapy services. Some models endorse using the same therapists in individual and family work while others do not support this approach. These models recommend referring the client out for the other therapy component or having a second therapist that is in house deliver the other component. While the approach of working both individually with the adolescent and with the family at the same time has advantages and is the approach chosen by CIFFTA, there are important pitfalls that you will want to consider, and therapists must be aware of what may go wrong when the same therapist conducts both individual and family sessions. Some therapists argue that the adolescent's independence is strengthened by having separate therapy and their own therapist. In CIFFTA we believe that the adolescent's independence is strengthened when the therapist helps the adolescent to be effective in becoming independent *and* helps the family to support and not constrain that independence. Linehan's DBT ascribes to the idea of having separate therapists in which a therapist delivers individual therapy, and a separate therapist focuses on the skills training component of the model (Linehan, 2014a, 2014b, in press-a, in press-b). Linehan asserts that it can be difficult for the individual therapist to be directive and to maintain focus on the didactic presentation of the skills as clients will want to draw the therapist to process recent events and crises, which can derail the skills training session (Linehan, 2014a, 2014b, in press-a, in press-b). We agree that this and similar challenges are real, and they must be identified and addressed if the same therapist attempts to work in two different modalities with the family.

An advantage of having the same therapist is that it allows you to understand the perspectives, needs, strengths, and challenges on both sides (i.e., adolescent and family), to watch how these interact in family sessions, and to facilitate interventions that will help each achieve their goals. In effect, it helps you to create the synergy between components that can be so powerful. For example, youth may need help communicating about certain topics with their family and caregivers, and family members may need help communicating with the youth. Furthermore, by reducing family conflict and strain, it makes it easier for the adolescent to engage in the process of healthy separation and individuation. By working together with both the adolescent individually and with the family, you can ease the stress and pressure within the family. When there are two therapists, it is much more difficult to maintain the same focus and to avoid having family process details fall through the cracks. It would take a lot of communication and organization to manage two therapists rather than one. The one-therapist approach is supported by CIFFTA so that there is synergy between the activities of the different components rather than cracks and gaps in communication and treatment strategies. The expectation is that the issues discussed in psychoeducational modules or individual therapy are followed up on at every opportunity in family therapy. We believe it is difficult for there to be optimal communication between multiple therapists working on such complex issues.

When implementing a model such as CIFFTA, in which you might be providing both family and individual therapy, *clarity and transparency about confidentiality are crucial.* Caregivers must know that it is not helpful if they ask the therapist for information about the youth that should remain confidential and that would lead to a reduction in the adolescent's trust of the therapist. On the other hand, you must know how to address an adolescent who seeks assurances that all information will be kept confidential, especially from their caregivers. When working with severe symptoms, it is critically important that you be clear about the limits in these areas. Beyond the usual legal limits (i.e., danger to self or others, child, or elderly abuse), you must discuss confidentiality regarding substance use and other self-harm behaviors. You cannot ensure total confidentiality regarding severe behaviors because any sustained deterioration that puts the adolescent in danger, or any sustained level of high use that suggests that the therapy is not helping, must be discussed with the caregiver(s). Within this model, it would be considered irresponsible and unethical on the part of the therapist to keep this type of information from a caregiver because it would undermine the protective functions family therapy should be promoting in them. We would be undercutting our own therapy values that convey the importance of protection in healthy families and the important role that caregivers play. As a therapist you cannot require more involved and effective parenting while simultaneously withholding information they need to protect the youth. The most you can ensure is that the confidentiality of adolescent information will be a top priority, and that if sensitive material must be discussed, the therapist will work hard to prepare both the youth and the caregivers to discuss the topics together and to respond in a productive and adaptive manner.

SUMMARY

In this chapter we presented a set of issues that can significantly impact the success of CIFFTA's implementation and effectiveness. We covered issues from the unique systemic characteristics of working with families to the selection and training of therapists, looking at competencies and abilities that are helpful to keep in mind. We also discussed a range of issues relevant to delivery of CIFFTA, including the frequency of sessions, ways of collecting data that can be used in tailoring treatment, and ending with unique issues in virtual and home-based delivery of services. We hope that this presentation allows therapists and agency leaders to think through how to prepare for successful implementation of CIFFTA or similar systemic family-based treatments.

5

CIFFTA Individual Therapy with the Adolescent

Individual therapy with the adolescent is one of CIFFTA's three main components. Not all family therapy models emphasize or even recommend individual work with the adolescent. Some family therapy treatments such as Brief Strategic Family Therapy (BSFT) choose to work exclusively with the conjoint family and do not include treatment components dedicated specifically to the adolescent (Szapocznik et al., 2012). The rationale behind BSFT's approach is that presenting symptoms are best handled through the family and the treatment model prescribes a sharp focus on family interactions and the role of the caregivers. The concern is that individual work with the adolescent can diffuse the focus of the therapy. Daniel A. Santisteban conducted a good amount of his early research on BSFT (Santisteban et al., 2003, 2006) but concluded that omitting a treatment component to facilitate the adolescent's journey toward an integrated, motivated, differentiated, and solidly connected self is a lost opportunity.

Within CIFFTA we find it beneficial to work with adolescents individually at the same time as you are working on family dynamics and interactions that facilitate or hinder healthy adolescent development (Santisteban et al., 2013). This approach takes advantage of the fact that adolescence is a developmental stage in which many significant changes are occurring, during which highly significant challenges are being navigated, and in which there are enormous opportunities for both individual and family growth. Both the individual and the family unit are challenged to grow and to become increasingly flexible, so it is powerful to work with both sides of the equation to bring about healthy change.

What should be avoided is for the individual therapy to *compete* with the family work for attention. The decision should never be to conduct individual work because it is hard to engage families. Individual work with adolescents must complement and create synergy with the family therapy work. For example, as the adolescent learns and develops skills, family sessions are the arena in which the youth begin to use the new skills. The family therapist helps family members to acknowledge and reinforce the positive changes being made by the adolescent. The therapist also identifies where the youth may go wrong in their delivery. In the other direction, the individual sessions can help an adolescent prepare for more effective family sessions, thinking through how new skills will make them more effective in the family context. Movement away from adolescent-family power struggles opens the door for an appreciation of all that families have to offer. This is the work of creating synergy between treatment components.

THE ADOLESCENT DEVELOPMENTAL STAGE AND IMPLICATIONS FOR TREATMENT

Adolescence can be divided into three developmental stages, early adolescence, middle adolescence, and late adolescence/young adulthood. While there is considerable agreement regarding the use of ages 10–13 to mark the beginning of early adolescence there is more debate regarding the upper limit. Typically, adolescence was thought to end at around age 18 but more recently there has been an emphasis on the *emerging adulthood* that extends to the early 20s. This extension focuses on the transition period into independent living and blurs the boundary between emerging adults and adolescents (Institute of Medicine and National Research Council, 2014). To understand the extraordinary changes that one finds within the adolescent developmental stage, the reader need only consider the significant differences between an 11-year-old youth and an 18-year-old. The differences in the biological, cognitive, psychosocial, and emotional domains are substantial and reflect the amount of change that is normative for this stage.

Because of the extraordinary changes occurring during adolescence, it is a critical time to modify risky behavior trajectories and to cultivate and sustain healthy habits. Abilities and behaviors that develop during adolescence are critical to long-term well-being. Identity development (e.g., race, ethnicity, gender identity, and sexual orientation), an understanding of one's place in the world, and an understanding of one's ability to impact the world (i.e., agency) begin to take shape. The search for autonomy and differentiation from caregivers begins and the ability to achieve differentiation while maintaining a strong and healthy connection is key. At times, healthy differentiation can be confused with physical and emotional disconnection, disengagement, and separation from caregivers and family members. Differentiation supported by family and occurring within the context of a strong relationship should be a therapeutic goal. There is consensus among experts that maintaining healthy relationships, emotional closeness, and open communication with caregivers and family members is essential during adolescence and can facilitate progress toward becoming an independent, well-functioning adult (Abrams, 2015).

During the adolescent stage, individuals begin to choose who they want to spend time with, and it is usually with peers. They take interest in making decisions for themselves related to sleep, exercise, eating habits, and substance use, as well as peer groups, romantic relationships, and educational and career paths. Part of the work is to begin to identify and differentiate wants from needs and to communicate these in a way that will make the youth effective at having their needs met. Adolescents begin to interact independently with adults and authority figures such as doctors, nurses, law enforcement, and school personnel. These steps mark the transition from childhood to adulthood, which if navigated in a healthy manner is a time of growth and great potential for youth.

Passage through the adolescent developmental stage is unique for each individual and there is much room for variation within the trajectory of each youth. Part of the variation is due to the surroundings or context (e.g., familial and societal) in which the youth is developing. For example, how much push back is there while the adolescent is struggling for independence? How much conflict, validation, and support are present in the family context? How much peer pressure toward risky behavior is the youth experiencing? What is the nature of their exposure to and participation in social media and technology and what is its impact? Is the adolescent confronting a great deal of discrimination, marginalization, economic hardship, exposure to violence, or conflicts around acculturation? Where is the adolescent in terms of sexual orientation, gender, race, and ethnic identity? Is there validation, rejection, or indifference regarding these aspects of their identity? When stressors begin to accumulate and overwhelm the capacity and resources of the adolescent, this increases the likelihood that youth's mental health and functioning will be negatively impacted.

Adolescence is a time when risky behaviors and mental disorders emerge (National Academies of Sciences, 2019a), so treatment should build resilience in adolescents as they encounter stressful situations and contexts. Treatment provides an opportunity for psychoeducation, prevention efforts, and for modifying a path from poor decision making, engagement in harmful behaviors, and negative outcomes to a constructive and healthy trajectory (Naar-King, 2011). There is no more critical time for treatment to ensure a healthy progression into adulthood.

CIFFTA INDIVIDUAL COMPONENT FOR THE ADOLESCENT

CIFFTA's major activities with the adolescent include (1) engaging and joining with the adolescent; (2) identification of, and tailoring treatment to cover, the most relevant and timely topics, stressors, and themes impacting the adolescent; (3) enhancing the adolescent's motivation to engage in treatment, process issues that are important to them, set healthy goals, and to make behavioral changes; (4) in-depth processing and generalization of the psychoeducation and skills information provided in psychoeducational sessions; (5) coaching the adolescent to effectively communicate in preparation for family interactions, especially family discussions around sensitive issues; and (6) monitoring risky behaviors, maintenance, and relapse prevention. Each of these sets of activities are described in more detail below.

Engaging and Joining the Adolescent

The early focus (pretreatment and the first several weeks) is to engage and join the adolescent. This sometimes includes validating their reluctance to participate in treatment. Many times, youth enter treatment because caregivers and other authority figures pressure them to attend treatment. In a real sense, the adolescent is not yet the therapist's *client* because they have not chosen to work with the therapist. This reality immediately puts the adolescent in a defensive position because to them, it feels as if they do not have a choice, and their autonomy has been stripped away by this process. If this is left unchanged, this stance is much more likely to lead to a power struggle than to a collaborative therapeutic relationship. When youth enter treatment as part of a diversion program or due to a transgression at school, therapy can also be perceived to be part of the "punishment" process for the transgressions.

In these situations, the therapist must help the adolescent to appreciate the true nature of the relationship between therapist and youth/

family as well as the relationship between therapist and the referring system (e.g., juvenile justice or school). In this early stage, the therapist cannot be perceived as rushing to make changes desired by the caregivers or the legal system and instead must take time to build trust and show genuine empathy for and interest in the youth. Confidentiality should be clearly discussed alone with the adolescent during this early phase. This helps build trust as they learn what to expect in terms of confidentiality and how the individual sessions will work jointly with the family sessions (more information on this complex issue is provided at the end of this chapter). The therapist should utilize engagement strategies to ensure that a strong alliance with the adolescent is formed. A useful way to start the first individual session is by saying something that sounds like "As you will see I am not here to tell you what you must do or how to do it. I am sure you have lots of people willing to do that. I am here to work together with you to find out what is important to you, what you want for your life, how you can be as effective as possible in getting those things you want, and how we can better align the goals you and your family have set. I am sorry if you feel you were pushed into this work, but if you are willing to continue, I would really like to see if I can help you meet your goals. Let me know what you think about this." This sets the stage for a collaborative process where the therapist and adolescent can cocreate goals for the individual work.

> ### Pointers for Early Stages of CIFFTA Individual Work
>
> - Get to know the adolescent in areas not related to "problems" and seek to understand and enhance their own intrinsic motivations to change.
> - Adolescents often come to therapy in a "one-down" position and are prepared to resist attempts to change them.
> - The therapist can be seen as no more than an "ally and agent" of the caregivers or outside institutions. The transition to making the adolescent a collaborator is crucially important.
> - A therapist is likely to fail if they seek major behavioral changes before enhancing motivation and aligning with the adolescent's agenda.

In some special cases, an adolescent may be powerful enough to resist entry into therapy, leaving caregivers completely frustrated

(Santisteban et al., 1994, 1996). For example, a caregiver may say that they are unable to bring the adolescent in because each time they go to school to pick up the adolescent to attend sessions, the adolescent fails to show up. Clearly in this scenario, the adolescent is a powerful figure who can thwart the caregiver's plans and wishes. It is particularly important in this scenario that the therapist reaches out to the adolescent directly and acknowledges that therapy can only work if it meets the adolescent's needs. The therapist seeks a direct relationship from the start that does not go "through" the caregiver who is powerless in relation to the youth. A therapist who is perceived as an ally of the weak caregivers against the powerful adolescent is a recipe for an unproductive and doomed power struggle. Therapists will lose this battle every time.

Therapists do well to be informed of what is happening in the lives of youth, social media, and in society so that they can have informed conversations about non-therapy–related issues. What may connect with an adolescent may be around sports, music, hobbies, or other events in the news. Some therapists find it helpful to have something interesting in their offices like magnetic darts and a dart board so that communication does not require staring into each other's eyes or faces. It is important to think through how to connect as people and not just as client and therapist. Too often therapy begins and never deviates away from talking about the presenting problems that brought the youth and family to treatment. This is less likely to succeed than taking some time to connect and to identify and discuss strengths that the youth possess. *Therapy is intimidating enough without jumping right into what is wrong with the youth and consistently maintaining a pathology and deficits focus.*

Identifying Themes to Work On with the Adolescent

In Chapter 4 we discussed the Tailoring Report and how it contributes to treatment planning by highlighting the most pressing adolescent needs, themes, and characteristics. Throughout the process of therapy, the CIFFTA therapist keeps their eyes and ears open to new emerging issues and continues to monitor changes in important aspects of adolescent functioning such as:

- Adolescent problem recognition and motivation to work toward healthy development.
- Adolescent problems such as depression, anxiety, impulsivity, substance use, self-harm, and involvement with the juvenile justice system.

- Working through the adolescent's ethnic and racial identity, sexual orientation, and gender identity, with the goal of supporting a healthy identity.
- Life skills that could be relevant during the adolescent developmental stage (e.g., interpersonal effectiveness, negotiating, decision making, emotion regulation, self-monitoring, more effective handling of social media, and coping skills).
- Monitoring peer pressure toward behavior problems.
- Monitoring problematic relationships and interactions with adults, peers, and institutions/systems.
- Identifying effective strategies for handling the stress resulting from discrimination, marginalization, and acculturation difficulties they experience.
- Identifying the presence of a traumatic event(s) and its impact.
- Being open to working with the family to cope with life stressors and to benefit from protective family factors.

The therapist must be attuned to the issues that are most significant and timely for the adolescent so that therapy can always be perceived as relevant, helpful, and ecologically valid. There is no shortage of complex struggles that adolescents are confronting for the very first time in their lives. Not even adolescents readily appreciate the complexity of this stage of development.

Enhancing Adolescent Motivation

Once the engagement phase is underway, the focus with the adolescent turns to enhancing adolescent motivation for change. Youngsters brought to treatment are often accustomed to being strongly confronted by adults in the family, school, legal, and treatment systems. Therapists must avoid falling into the trap of being perceived as one more confronting adult that is pushing the adolescent to be someone they are not. Early work should incorporate evidence-based interventions designed to create a collaborative relationship with adolescents and help them develop their own goals and intrinsic motivation for change without triggering the defensive behavior that confrontation tends to elicit. The growing evidence demonstrating MI's success in working without creating resistance (Miller & Rollnick, 2023) and the ease with which it can be combined with other treatments make it an integral component of adolescent treatment and led to its integration into CIFFTA's work.

An early step is to evaluate the stage of change the adolescent is currently in. Does the adolescent feel that there is a problem with the behavior and/or symptom identified as the presenting issue(s) or do they think it is no big deal? Do they think there may be a problem, but it is too hard to change and not worth the effort? The stage-of-change work by Prochaska and DiClemente (1992) is invaluable in this effort.

> ### *The Stages of Change*
>
> - **Precontemplation:** Not yet acknowledging that there is a problem behavior that needs to be changed
> - **Contemplation:** Acknowledging that there is a problem but not yet ready or sure of wanting to make a change
> - **Preparation:** Getting ready to change
> - **Action:** Changing behavior
> - **Maintenance:** Maintaining the behavior change
> - **Relapse:** Returning to older behaviors and abandoning the new changes

The stages of change are used to better understand whether the adolescent is in precontemplation, contemplation, preparation, action, or maintenance. This allows the therapist to select the appropriate strategies to explore and identify goals, build motivation for change within the adolescent, and help the adolescent devise a realistic plan for change. If a therapist interacts with an adolescent who is in precontemplation (i.e., an adolescent that does not acknowledge the existence of a problem) but attempts to use strategies designed for a person who is prepared to make substantial changes in an acknowledged problem, the therapist will likely lose the adolescent and erode the alliance they worked so hard to establish.

The goal is to work with the adolescent to increase their awareness of a need for change and the motivation to participate in treatment, and then assist the adolescent in selecting targets and methods for change. This type of work cannot be rushed. It must go at a pace that fits the adolescent's situation and circumstances. One of the most common mistakes made by therapists is to rush through this work in an attempt to get to the change phase more quickly. But when this process is rushed, change attempts fail and failure can lead to frustration for both parties. Once the tone of collaboration has been set, the therapist moves toward setting an agenda that is driven in large part by the adolescent. This work includes eliciting the adolescent's honest view of their current situation and whether their lives have been complicated by the presenting problems. They can also honestly consider potential goals for their life. These goals must be separate from the goals of caregivers, which at the initiation of therapy are usually more about behavior control. A major goal is to achieve an alignment of healthy adolescent and family goals. Although we are focusing on the youth's needs and goals here, it is obviously unrealistic to go too far into treatment while downplaying the needs and expectations of the family. MI is designed to nurture the youth's own creation of goals and reasons for behavior change and then work to align them with the family's goals for the adolescent's well-being. Expressing empathy and taking the time to evoke the adolescent's perspective is a collaborative process that supports autonomy and emphasizes the spirit of MI.

During motivation enhancement work, the adolescent shares what is occurring in their life, what is important to them, and what areas they want to focus on. The driving force is *within* them rather than external (i.e., caregivers, school, therapist, and courts). Collaboratively setting the adolescent's goals ensures that they perceive therapy as helpful with their personal and normative struggles. Sometimes the therapist may be surprised by the reason or motivation for change that the adolescent discovers and communicates and why the effort is worthwhile. The therapist encourages the emergence and amplification of discrepancies between present behavior and short- and long-term goals. The emergence of the adolescent's ambivalence is an important step, and the ambivalence needs to be amplified during the change process. Ambivalence is normal and expected, however, if it is not resolved, it can slow or halt progress. The ultimate goal in MI is to assist the youth in resolving their ambivalence and to collaborate with them as they increase their motivation to change and grow. Early work on ambivalence does not mean it will not resurface. Even when someone wants to make changes or starts to make positive changes, ambivalence can continue to be present. Clinicians do well to normalize the experience of ambivalence and empathize with the process.

Engaging with the youth in the spirit of MI means that the therapist supports the development of autonomy in the youth, which is also an important developmental task of adolescence. Providing the opportunity in the individual sessions for the youth to make decisions and share thoughts and feelings fosters critical thinking, introspection, and autonomy. The therapist avoids "pushing" the adolescent to change, giving too much advice, or prematurely focusing on fixing the problems. This would only lead the adolescent to shut down, rebel, and create discord between the therapist and the youth.

Examples of Confrontational Messages to Avoid

- "You are really hurting your caregivers by behaving so badly."
- "You do realize that you won't get into college with these types of grades."
- "Why don't you stop using marijuana? If you really wanted to and could, you would."
- "You are depressed, and your drinking makes it worse. You aren't going to feel better by using. Isn't it better to just stop?"

Utilization of the principles of MI (e.g., express empathy, develop discrepancy, support self-efficacy) along with the MI skills (OARS: open-ended questions, affirmations, reflections, and summaries) supports the resolution of ambivalence, a reduction in adolescent speech that sustains the problem behavior, and the eliciting of talk that indicates readiness for change (Naar-King, 2011). When an adolescent is on board with making a change, individual sessions are used to help the adolescent establish life goals that will lead them to a healthier life.

It is important to be curious about discrepancies and to maintain a nonjudgmental stance, avoiding anything that sounds like a *gotcha* moment. A therapist may use linking phrases, such as "on the one hand" and "on the other hand," to help the adolescent acknowledge conflicting statements without aggressively confronting the inconsistencies. Linking summaries creates an opportunity in the conversation that highlights conflicting ideas or discrepancies that help the adolescent to acknowledge and address the discrepancy or topic without feeling confronted or put down. MI helps the therapist to be aware of the unwanted reactions and discord that any statement may elicit. A great example is when the therapist asks the client something like "On a scale from 1 to 10, how important do you think it is to change your drinking behavior?" If the client says 5, a common therapist response might be "Really, I would have said a 7 based on what you have told me and the problems that brought you here. Why just a 5?" The adolescent response that this therapist statement might elicit would be to generate all the reasons why the problem is not as bad as a 7. Is that really the position the therapist would want the adolescent to take? The effective MI therapist would say, "Oh really, a 5, why did you choose that number and not a 2?" By asking the question in this way, the therapist encourages the adolescent to honestly connect with the reasons why the problem drinking is more problematic than a 2. Most importantly, they would be *the adolescent's reasons* and no one else's.

In-Depth Processing of Key Themes

Individual therapy is the place to allow adolescents to explore and work through issues that they find difficult to address with peers, teachers, and particularly with family members. Once discussions of sensitive topics have led to conflict in families, it takes considerable skill to change the habitual interaction the next time that same topic is discussed. The CIFFTA therapist has the opportunity to explore issues that are important to the adolescent and that they may not typically discuss with others. Examples include ethnic/racial identity, being the victim of bullying, being the targets of racism/discrimination, sexual orientation or gender identity, and having problems relating to peers. The youth can also share their concern regarding family situations such as family members misusing substances, financial issues, parental conflict, or family members at risk of being deported or incarcerated. The therapist actively works with the adolescent so that they can clarify their own view on the matter, and then, when appropriate, encourages and prepares the adolescent to discuss these issues effectively with other family members, preferably in CIFFTA family therapy sessions. The adolescent may be struggling with the fact that they do not feel that they belong to any particular group. They may feel that they are not sure about their sexual orientation or that their orientation is not supported by peers and loved ones. They may not feel that they are a part of the host culture, or they might feel that they belong to the host culture, but the caregivers don't. These types of issues can impact the level of trust, acceptance, and connection the adolescent feels with peers, caregivers, and other loved ones. All of these situations place strain on the adolescent and on caregiver–adolescent relationships. An important task for the therapist is to process these issues with the adolescent to help them feel comfort in their own skin and to make decisions about whether to communicate more deeply about these issues with peers and family. The therapist must help adolescents to challenge any internalized oppression that prevents them from feeling comfortable with their decision.

Working with LGBTQ+ Youth

In our individual work with adolescents over the years, we worked with LGBTQ+ youth as a natural part of the therapy and made no specific systematic adjustments to the work. But as we extended our work to treat self-harm and suicide-related behavior, we found that LGBTQ+

youth were disproportionately overrepresented in the population (Mena et al., 2024a). Our experience was consistent with a 2019 survey that found that an alarming 46.8% of LGBTQ+ youth had seriously considered attempting suicide, 40.2% had made a suicide plan, and 23.4% had attempted suicide (Ivey-Stephenson et al., 2020). The elevated risk is increased exponentially by the fact that LGBTQ+ youth are also five times more likely to use alcohol and drugs than their heterosexual peers (Goldbach & Gibbs, 2015; Centers for Disease Control and Prevention, 2016). Substance misuse can be a natural consequence of the chronic stressors they experience and can also exacerbate or trigger self-harm behavior. We realized how important it was for us to make this set of risks better known to therapists working with youth.

As a result of our experiences and findings, we began to take a more structured and systematic approach to addressing the types of stressors and key issues LGBTQ+ youth typically brought to treatment and created psychoeducational modules to address them. This included emphasizing how being both a racial/ethnic minority and a sexual and gender minority can result in a compounding set of adverse outcomes (Cyrus, 2017). Intersectionality highlights the importance of considering racial, ethnic, and sexual and gender minority status as deeply interconnected, rather than distinct experiences (Rosenthal, 2016). LGBTQ+ youth of color can experience racism from society as well as from within the LGBTQ+ community (Hailey et al., 2020) and homophobia and transphobia in the society in general and within the community of color. Compared with White LGBTQ+ youth, Latine LGBTQ+ youth were found to be even more likely to attempt suicide (Bostwick et al., 2014). Mueller et al. (2015) found that "Black LGB youths were more likely than their White heterosexual same-gender peers to report suicide ideation" (p. 983). LGBTQ+ Latine and Black youth may experience more difficulties in the process of coming out, in obtaining caregiver and family support, and in the extent to which they feel a sense of belonging in their community when compared to non-Latine White LGBTQ+ youth (Human Rights Campaign, 2012).

Goldbach and Gibbs (2015) use Minority Stress theory to understand the possible contribution of both distal and proximal factors. Among the significant *distal factors,* these researchers found that living at home and being in school were both associated with less marijuana use while greater experiences of violence/victimization and having come out to more people were related to increased psychological distress. The increased stress due to having more people aware of the youth's sexual orientation is particularly problematic if it is connected to increased marginalization and victimization. Among the significant *proximal* factors, Goldbach and Gibbs (2015) found that internalized homophobia, defined as negative feelings about the identification as gay or lesbian, was associated with marijuana use. Connectedness to the gay community was generally associated with lower internalized homophobia. This is a particularly interesting dynamic to understand given that there have been reports of higher substance use in this same community, due to more permissive norms regarding substance use. In this latter example, community connectedness might be considered protective because of its link to lower internalized homophobia but a risk when the community contributes to increasing substance use.

Some of the enhancements that we made for LGBTQ+ youth reporting self-harm behavior were more focused on the self-harm dimensions and would be used even with non-LGBTQ+ youth. These include enhancements focused on emotion dysregulation, poor interpersonal skills, educating youth and caregivers about self-harm and the intrapersonal and interpersonal triggers to self-harm, and the many co-occurring mental health-related conditions (e.g., depression and substance misuse) that can exacerbate symptoms and complicate treatment.

When working individually with LGBTQ+ adolescents, CIFFTA therapists are trained to discuss disclosure. Specifically, you must think about how to discuss the options of disclosure with adolescents who have not disclosed to caregivers or who have disclosed only to some family members and peers. It is important for the therapist to have up-to-date information and talking points regarding the pros and cons of disclosure, and how the quality of the relationship prior to any disclosure can determine the family member's response. It should not be assumed that immediate disclosure, or any disclosure, is the best route in all circumstances—this is an important decision point for the youth. Goldbach and Gibbs (2015) found that premature disclosure and/or disclosure to the wrong people can increase the likelihood of victimization. The therapist can help the youth make an informed decision on the next steps they would like to take. During individual work with the adolescent, it is also important to validate the frustrations they feel regarding peers, family members, and systems that are nonaffirming while at the same time working with the adolescent to be resilient and to succeed in these contexts. The balance between change and acceptance of contexts that are slow to change is always an important part of the therapeutic process.

Working with Youth as They Develop a Race and Ethnic Identity

The development of an ethnic and racial identity is another key task for a Latine youth during the adolescent developmental stage. The process involves not only labeling oneself but feeling a part of a group. Although there is much conversation about whether race and ethnic identity should be distinct, there tends to be a blurry line between race and ethnicity, and it typically is difficult to distinguish the two for many of the people we work with. One solution is to allow the identity to be integrated in whatever way the youth choose. The term *ethnic and racial identity* has been coined as a way of talking about an integrated identity that refers to the "experiences that reflect both individuals' ethnic background and their racialized experience as a member of a particular group in the context of the United States" (Umaña-Taylor et al., 2014, p. 23). Although this process of identity formation is active during the adolescent stage, it should not be thought of as static or occurring only during these years. Ethnic and racial identity is constantly evolving throughout the different life cycle stages. This is impacted not only by maturation but also by the changing contexts in which the individual finds themselves. In different contexts there will be attitudes they confront (e.g., racism and anti-immigrant sentiment) that have a strong influence on identity. The process of attaching meaning to one's identity can be fueled by experiences of racism and discrimination. Meaning also emerges from active participation in activities that help them explore identity or connect to people who share their identity. Positive regard and affirmation are important in determining the pride that an individual can feel, and this ultimately can be linked to well-being and healthy development and behaviors (Castro et al., 2009). A therapist working with Latine youth must be able to discuss this complex process and support the youth as they explore, share positive and negative feelings regarding their identities, and consider the extent to which external messages have been internalized.

Generalizing Module Material

For key themes that often surface during the adolescent stage, such as self-harm, substance use, social media processes, risky sexual behavior, or other unique stressors, we have psychoeducational material (described fully in Chapter 7) that can provide the foundation of knowledge and skills to better address the issues. Following the delivery of the module, the subsequent individual sessions focus on applying the information and skills to their life and unique circumstances. The therapist provides a space in which the adolescent can discuss their thoughts, feelings, and concerns about how and when to use skills and new information. For example, if the youth learned about interpersonal effectiveness skills, they learned how to identify needs and how to communicate these needs to significant others in a way and at a time that is more likely to get the needs met. Guidance on how to successfully use this in everyday situations is the focus of generalization work. In individual sessions, the therapist helps the adolescent report on when the skills worked, when they didn't, and how the implementation of the skills may have to be tweaked to make them more useful and effective. The situation they describe may be in school, with peers, or with family members. When the context in which the skill was tried is the family, individual sessions can be used to refine the delivery, and the next family session may be used as an *in vivo* opportunity to try out the skill. In the family session, the therapist helps to shape the adolescent's delivery as well as the family's response to the adolescent. An analysis of the moment and the way that the adolescent attempted to use the skill may show that it was not used correctly or that it can be refined to increase its effectiveness. It can also show that family members are not responding effectively and that a rigid and maladaptive family response also needs to be tweaked. The same may be true for material learned regarding acculturation and acculturation stress, blended family issues, and many other module themes.

In the case of Juan and his mother (who we describe in more detail in Chapter 8), the youngster was having difficulty managing his anger and had emotional outbursts regularly. The anger was in part due to feeling his needs were not met or even acknowledged. The interpersonal effectiveness skills helped Juan learn strategies for communicating in an assertive not aggressive manner and to avoid rupturing relationships due to the way he expressed himself with others. Emotion regulation was also helpful. In the individual therapy session with Juan that followed completion of the module, the therapist focused on generalizing skills that were learned to specific situations in Juan's daily life. He was able to identify his anger earlier (before reacting in a maladaptive manner) and make better decisions about what to do to soothe himself without bringing harm to himself or his relationships. They also practiced how he would use the interpersonal effectiveness skills with his mother.

In the case of Maria (who we will also describe in more detail in Chapter 8), the distress tolerance module was prioritized. In individual sessions Maria shared that she needed to control her emotions and manage her reactions because she did not want to lose her relationships. In the individual sessions with Maria following completion of the module, the therapist focused on generalizing the distress tolerance skills by helping Maria create a plan for tolerating distress. This included strategies (e.g., using a grounding technique and journaling) that Maria agreed she could implement when her emotions were intense. This would help her tolerate the moment, allow the emotion to subside, and keep her from damaging relationships that were important to her. In later sessions, the distress tolerance skills that were learned were generalized to other areas of Maria's life and situations. These included difficult interactions with peers and her mother.

Coaching Adolescents to Promote Successful Family Discussions

Families have deeply entrenched patterns of relating to each other that are difficult to change, and it may be particularly difficult to change behavior and perspectives as they relate to sensitive issues such as substance use, risky sexual behavior, sexual orientation, and gender identity. Therapists use every tool in the CIFFTA toolbox to decrease rigid, hostile, and conflictual family interactions and to increase validating and supportive family interactions. To achieve these, the CIFFTA family and individual sessions work together. When the therapist identifies a habitual interaction within the family that they wish to change, the therapist may decide that it would be effective to prepare and coach the adolescent in individual sessions to behave in a way (in family sessions) that is likely to change the family interaction to a more successful and adaptive one.

When an adolescent has been using substances and/or having problems at school, with peers, or with the legal system, it is common to see a pattern of interaction in which caregivers are angry and have little patience. They tend to criticize and invalidate the adolescent. The adolescent tends to go into the interaction angry and prepared for battle rather than calmly and prepared to interact in a new more effective way. To better handle these difficult situations, the therapist prepares the adolescent to anticipate recurring patterns that trap them into the habitual negative responses and to break the pattern with a different response. Coaching is key to making this successful, and the therapist may ask the adolescent to practice using role plays in individual sessions. These processes serve two main purposes. One is to help improve the relationship between the adolescent and their family. A second purpose is to help the adolescent develop a sense of self-efficacy and power in that they can successfully handle and negotiate difficult relationship problems. These changes help them be more effective with other important relations as well, such as with teachers and peers.

Monitoring Risky Behaviors, Maintenance, and Relapse Prevention

Behaviors such as recurring substance use, self-harm, and other risky behaviors that put the youth's life at risk, must be monitored during individual sessions. These types of behaviors are not only largely concealed in conjoint sessions, but they might sometimes be overshadowed by the intensity of family sessions. It can also become counterproductive if the family sessions become overly focused on monitoring the risky behavior(s) and disregard the need to change important family processes such as validation, communication, and parenting.

When discussing maladaptive behaviors in individual sessions, it may become obvious that adolescents have trouble connecting the dots on problem behaviors, emotional states, and other possible triggers. As originally designed by Linehan (1993) and others, the use of diary cards facilitate the identification and analysis of emotional events, intrapersonal and interpersonal triggers to behaviors that are concerning, urges and impulses, and the use of skills to help break the sequence between triggers, urges, and problem behaviors such as self-harm or substance use. The identification of the trigger and the maladaptive behavior helps find the exact place in the sequence where a new skill can help to weaken the power of the urge to elicit the undesirable outcome. Diary cards can play an important role in treatment, but they must be done in a way that is feasible and acceptable to the youth given that actual completion of the diary is always the main challenge.

Reducing Self-Harm Behavior Using Diary Cards and Skills

During individual sessions with Maria, the therapist monitored her self-harm behavior using the diary card and documented when cutting behavior had occurred. This helped identify possible triggers to self-harm behaviors. The therapist reinforced the use of the distress tolerance plan that had been established while completing the psychoeducation module. Halfway through treatment, Maria had stopped cutting.

Individual sessions are a venue that give the adolescent a space to be honest about their struggles with risky behaviors (e.g., self-harm, increased substance use, skipping school, risky sexual behavior) without worrying that family members were not prepared to hear it and would react poorly. And yet the therapist is always aware that the family is in some ways being deprived of information that it needs to protect the youth. If families remain unaware of the youth's risky behaviors and if the risky behaviors are not decreasing, we are not helping the family to protect the youth. For this reason, it becomes an important therapeutic goal to work with adolescents so they can disclose information about their risky behaviors to the family. As adolescents change their perspective on risky behaviors and can communicate that it is a problem that they want to change, they can more readily speak about it openly with the family and begin to receive support and guidance in their struggle or change attempts. The therapist's ability to assist the youth on how to communicate effectively with caregivers regarding risky behaviors is key.

In the late stage of treatment, the focus shifts to maintenance of behavior changes made and relapse prevention. Remember that some form of slip or relapse should typically be expected and the extent to which the youth is prepared for relapses may determine how well they manage the moment, maintain hope, and focus on getting back on track. During the individual sessions, the therapist takes time to check in with the adolescent on how things are progressing both individually and within the family. Special attention is paid to triggers to behaviors such as substance use, impulsivity, and conflictual family interactions. Barriers to maintaining change and solutions are discussed. The therapist and the youth must remain open to modifying the plan when relapses occur. But most often, what is needed is to reinforce the strategies that worked in treatment and to acknowledge how the adolescent may have deviated from those things that had been successful. Finally, when appropriate, the therapist works with the youth to engage in the discussion of relapse during family sessions. In the case of Ramon, relapse prevention was addressed by encouraging Ramon to share his progress, triggers, and barriers with his mother during family sessions. This openness allowed the mother the opportunity to express her love, caring, and support of him and to understand his vulnerabilities and stressors. She was able to let him know that he did not need to feel shame about urges to use and that they could use the power of the family to reduce slips and lapses.

Adjusting to Individual Variability within the Developmental Stage

CIFFTA treats adolescents who are of different ages and in different places along the developmental continuum so the challenges they face may be quite different. The focus of CIFFTA is primarily on adolescents ages 10–18, but we acknowledge that many of the issues we address continue to be highly relevant to the late adolescence/young adulthood stage (18–21 and beyond). The CIFFTA individual component can be tailored to account for these developmental differences in youth. For example, younger, less mature adolescents who are 10 or 12 years old may not benefit as much from certain aspects of the CIFFTA individual component, such as MI. They may benefit from more frequent family sessions, being more receptive to certain parenting interventions, and learning skills related to emotion regulation. Youth who are introspective or who show risky behaviors over an extended period, may benefit more from MI. As they are farther along in age and expected to make more decisions on their own, there may be more opportunities for individual work and a focus on the skills needed to meet those challenges effectively.

CIFFTA's modular approach is designed to address variability in symptoms. Youth who are showing early signs of vulnerability, such as depressive symptoms, behavioral issues, academic problems, peer difficulties, and/or familial conflict have different treatment needs than youth who are making daily choices to turn to drugs and other struggling peers to cope with emotional turmoil and/or life stressors. The flexibility of the CIFFTA individual component allows the therapist to select the focus of the individual sessions that will make the treatment most relevant for the youth and lead to the best possible outcomes.

Processing Issues of Confidentiality

Remember to address the issue of confidentiality very carefully with adolescents and caregivers (as described in Chapter 4). It is often effective to begin the conversation about confidentiality together with the caregivers and youth present so that everyone is clear and on the same page regarding the limits of confidentiality. Although this is most important as therapy begins, this is one of those issues that must be discussed and renegotiated throughout the process of therapy as new issues emerge and as the therapist decides whether risky behaviors are improving, deteriorating, or remaining unchanged. If not handled carefully and in a totally transparent fashion, a disagreement around confidentiality can erode the trust that is needed for therapy to be successful.

Staying on Track

The CIFFTA Treatment Plan and the CIFFTA Postsession Therapist Self-Report of Adherence are designed to help you stay on track as you plan adolescent interventions and reflect on what was delivered in session. Below are examples of questions that therapists can ask themselves while engaging in the individual work with the adolescent. The questions can keep the therapy focused and on track.

- "Did I engage the adolescent around issues that are not 'problem' related?"
- "Do I feel that we have established a collaborative relationship in which there is trust?"
- "Did I work to elicit and increase the adolescent's unique motivation to change?"
- "Did I make the adolescent feel comfortable with the idea of

therapy and ensure I am not seen as an adversary, or merely an 'ally of a punishing system'?"
- "Do I have a good handle on the unique themes the adolescent can benefit from addressing in therapy?"
- "Do I have an understanding of the environmental stressors the adolescent must live with and how these can best be addressed?"
- "Do I have a good sense of the skills that would help them with things like emotion regulation and interpersonal effectiveness and did I help in these areas using modules?"
- "Have I focused on how to ensure effective generalization of what they have learned to their daily lives?"
- "Did I identify knowledge and skills gaps and help by providing information modules?"
- "Do I have a good understanding of the adolescent's comfort with their identity (race, ethnicity, sexual orientation, and gender) and help them explore these issues in a supportive and affirming context?"
- "Did I help the adolescent develop and practice new behaviors that will make family interactions more open, honest, and supportive?"

SUMMARY

In this chapter we presented the key steps in integrating an individually focused component within the CIFFTA model and the goals for implementing the individual sessions effectively. We talked about the importance of the adolescent developmental stage and how many of the unique challenges that emerge can be seamlessly integrated into the therapy agenda and treatment plan. In this chapter we also highlighted some of the main tasks for the therapist such as monitoring risky behavior and enhancing motivation. We showed how individual work can be used to complement other CIFFTA components so that they work together to achieve the goals of the family. For example, the CIFFTA therapist must always keep in mind how the individual and family sessions are working in a synergistic fashion to meet both adolescent and family goals.

6

CIFFTA Therapy with the Entire Family

There is a growing appreciation for the importance of *family involvement* in almost any treatment that involves children and youth. This is true even when the meaning of that phrase is not well articulated. There is a continuum of what family involvement can entail. In Chapter 4, we presented a systematic way of thinking about the different levels of family work (Doherty, 1995). Even treatments that are often characterized as focusing on the individual, such as Trauma-Focused Cognitive-Behavioral Therapy (TF-CBT), include substantial family and caregiver components. This is the result of an appreciation for the power of the family context, whether it be in the role of promoting healing or creating risk. As we noted in Chapter 1, it is important to remember that there are many types of "families" and that blood relatives are not the only significant persons that end up being considered "like family" and have the potential to impact well-being.

The family is the space in which children are socialized, grow, and develop physically and emotionally. In the family, children learn how to maintain and deepen relationships with others, establish values, develop an identity, and learn about culturally defined ways of being, even when the values are not taught overtly. As children move through their developmental stages, so does the family move through predictable life cycle stages and each stage brings with it unique challenges and rewards (Carter & McGoldrick, 1999). Some families *flex and adapt* to better handle new circumstances and challenges and some families become rigid and struggle. Flexibility is key to good family functioning because it allows for new adjustments and solutions to be incorporated into the family to meet emerging conditions. By helping the family find new solutions, the therapist increases family flexibility.

The CIFFTA therapists observe *in vivo* family interactions to understand the forces that are supporting or constraining the adjustments the family must make in emerging conditions. At any given time when an individual is struggling with symptoms or problem behaviors, there are often systemic and relational influences that are maintaining problem behaviors or constraining solutions. Communications that constrain can be as simple as "This is not the way we do things in our family." The message is not always communicated openly but can be communicated in subtle and indirect ways. Other subtle but maladaptive relational interactions can constitute the fertile ground in which problems can take root and be maintained. One example of how a family system can maintain a problem was identified by Patterson (1982) and labeled *Coercive Family Processes*. In these interactions, the response from a family system to child or adolescent misbehavior can unwittingly reinforce the problem behavior and make it more likely to continue. For example, if a parent's nagging of the child ends only when the child explodes and throws things around the house, then the explosive behavior is reinforced. The behavior is reinforced because the nagging stops when the explosive behavior emerges and is shown to have power. When families enter treatment, therapists look to modify these maladaptive relational patterns at the same time as they mobilize family processes that can serve a protective role. These protective processes are key to buffering youth and other family members from outside stressors such as discrimination and racism.

In this chapter we present details on relational and systemic goals and interventions used within the family component of CIFFTA. As we train therapists to deliver CIFFTA's family treatment component, we focus on four major competencies: (1) systemic conceptualization of the presenting problem(s) and family functioning, (2) engagement of family members who are reluctant to participate in treatment and the thorough joining of all family members, (3) seeing and discerning the family process (or family dance, as Salvador Minuchin called it), and (4) the techniques used to modify the family relationships and interactions and that create greater support and decrease conflict and constraint. In the next section we present more detail on the targets of family interventions, the interventions themselves, and the competencies that the family therapist must master to deliver CIFFTA effectively.

SYSTEMIC CONCEPTUALIZATION

The first task for a family therapist with a new family is to look past the identification of individual-level presenting problems and histories, to a relational and systemic conceptualization of the presenting problem(s). Fishman (2022) sees this as one of the foundational competencies that a therapist must develop if they are going to be successful in family therapy. He describes family context as capable of "triggering certain characteristics within the individual, while causing others to become unattended and psychologically unimportant." When families are struggling, family forces may become relational triggers to problem behaviors. At the same time these same forces may cause positive, loving, and caring aspects of the individual to be dismissed or buried in the avalanche of negativity. It is not that these positive characteristics disappear, it is more that they are being constrained and hidden by the downward spiral in the family.

To give an example of how contextual factors work, consider how we process co-existing images in Rubin's vase, in which one must zoom in and out to focus on different aspects of the image. The intentional act of adjusting our attention and zooming in and out allows us to see different realities. Depending on how we process the border of black and white, we may see an elaborate cup in black or two faces facing each other in white. As we look at Figure 6.1, we can consciously shift our focus toward seeing a vase or seeing faces.

Likewise, in therapy you can zoom in and out of individual and larger systemic and relational aspects to capture the full reality of a behavior and to reveal new treatment options. If explosive behavior is simply maintained by emotion dysregulation or impulsivity, then

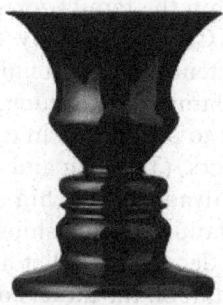

FIGURE 6.1. Rubin's vase.

changing these underlying factors is the only treatment option you have. But if there is a systemic contribution to the problem as well, then you can also modify the behavior by modifying the systemic and relational influences. Your options for treatment are multiplied. Think about the Patterson coercive process we discussed above to think about how relational factors can maintain a problem and how you can modify that sequence to help change the youth's explosive behavior. Rather than only focus on adolescent intrapersonal factors such as possible emotion dysregulation, the therapist can focus on triggers such as "nagging" and reinforcers such as giving the adolescent what they want only if and when they explode. It does not mean you cannot work with factors within the adolescent, just that you have more paths for treatment. Is a young person who is fighting often with peers simply aggressive and suffering from emotion dysregulation? Does it make a difference that when we look past the individual, we see that he lives in a dangerous neighborhood in which he feels unprotected and that he must make sure others perceive him as strong and tough if he is to survive? Perhaps both are true, but it would be irresponsible to ignore the external forces that require his toughness and even aggression. Furthermore, it may be possible to reduce aggressive behavior by working on impulsivity, changing the dangerous context, or better yet working on both simultaneously.

It is also helpful to families when they become more aware of contextual and relational impacts. Many families are unaware of the profound impact of the chronic stressors the youth are experiencing (e.g., poorly performing schools, racism and marginalization, risky neighborhoods). A therapist may say, "I know that it does not excuse your daughter's behavior, but it certainly rings true that there may be some level of unfairness in the way school staff hold some kids responsible and not others for the same behavior. I can also imagine how that can lead to additional frustration. I wonder if we should hear a bit more from your daughter and determine if it is worth exploring this?" In the same way, you would do well to consider what is happening in the caregiver world and context to better understand their behavior and their frustrations. A systemic formulation helps you to understand that when a caregiver is being intimidated at work, passed over for promotions, or receiving cuts in pay or in work hours, these stresses can negatively impact caregiver and parenting behavior. In summary, the ability to find more contributing factors in the client's context reveals more complexity in the clinical situation and gives the client and the therapist more treatment options. Just the act of having you validate the family member's experiences can go a long way to achieving a therapeutic impact.

ENGAGING AND JOINING THE FAMILY

Family therapy works only if we successfully engage in treatment, all family members who are needed to make treatment successful. Despite the importance of family member engagement, it has received much less attention than other intervention components. This has led to frustration among service providers who have the desire to work with families but can never really get the process off the ground. Furthermore, attempts to turn to home-based therapy as a way of solving the engagement problem have hit its own brick walls because going to the home brings its own complexities and problems. Going to the home does not guarantee that the key family members will be home even if they are scheduled, and there are many additional distractions that can hinder treatment impact. To be successful, the family therapist must have the knowledge, attitude, and skills necessary to mobilize the system toward engagement. CIFFTA has made engagement and joining (Santisteban & Szapocznik, 1994; Szapocznik et al., 1988) a key competency that is the focus of training and coaching. It is revealing that of all our publications, the work on engagement has been the most cited and used information in the field.

Once the family is in the therapy room, building a strong therapeutic alliance requires getting to know the family and its history, fully engaging, and joining each family member, building trust, hope, and credibility with the family, and enhancing the family's readiness for change. The early phase of treatment focuses on the engagement and joining work and may be the main focus of the first several sessions or longer depending on the family. Of course, to some extent this work continues throughout the entire course of treatment. Sometimes joining family members once they are in the therapy room is straightforward. You can get to know individuals in a way that is not merely about the presenting problem that they seek to address. Getting to know an adolescent's interests, hobbies, likes, and dislikes is important before beginning to hear complaints about the youth's behavior.

The more difficult phase is often what is happening prior to the family attending a session. To be truly effective you must widen the engagement lens to focus on the clinical and family dynamics that emerge from the very first phone call to a clinic, agency, or therapist. An interesting problem during the first phase of treatment is that while it is typically easier to engage and bring some family members to therapy, it is often the family member(s) that is more difficult to engage that can bring about the most change in the family condition (Santisteban & Szapocznik, 1994). The reluctance to come to therapy is often a red flag that the person is isolated and/or in conflict within the family system. When a father is fed up and has given up on his daughter, that is a family process that must be changed but it may also lead him to refuse to attend therapy. If we bring to treatment only the family members that come in easily, then we leave out people, and processes, that are keys to success in therapy. It is important that the therapist not rush the process of engagement because getting off to a good start with the right people in the session is central to success.

Challenging the Term *Resistance* and Better Understanding *Reluctance* to Enter Therapy

When clients are unsure about engaging in a treatment process and later in a treatment plan, we often label them as *resistant* because "they won't follow through the way they should." The *resistant client* is defined as the client who does not readily comply with the expert directives to come to treatment or to follow the treatment plan. The resistance label lays responsibility totally on the client and removes responsibility from the mental health specialist who may be pushing a client prematurely into a therapeutic situation and change. As we showed in Chapter 5 in the section on MI, commonly used therapy approaches can create the very resistance we don't want to encounter. The term *resistance* allows us to move forward without questioning how we approached the family or the fit between an intervention and the client's needs and preferences. It assumes that of course everyone will agree with the characteristics and assumptions of the treatment that we as therapists have selected. Too often we fail to question the processes and goals we have developed without client input. Next time you have a get together of family or friends, try to push someone toward the living room without explanation. You will detect resistance as they seek to stay standing straight in the same position they had. Try instead to tell them you want to show them something they will love in the living room and see if the reaction is any different. We as therapists help to create the context and meaning of therapy, and we should not take that responsibility for granted.

Let's consider the simple act of understanding how the family was referred to treatment. Unless a family is self-referred, there may be entities outside of the family that are pushing or "strongly recommending" counseling for the child or adolescent. When the family is feeling even slightly *forced or coerced* into treatment, the therapist can be initially perceived as an extension of the coercive and intrusive system. For example, if a family is referred by the juvenile justice system and the youth and family sees this as part of the punishment for the youth's transgression, then the therapist can easily be seen as an extension of the punishment system *and therapy is perceived as an integral part of the punishment experience*. The first task for the therapist in this situation is to acknowledge these forces and meanings, to differentiate themselves from that perceived coercive system, to acknowledge that it does not feel good to be pushed into treatment, and to help the family process their reaction to the pressure. Therapists must challenge their own conceptualizations of terms such as *resistance* and acknowledge that there may be some very healthy reasons (e.g., bad experiences with treatment and/or poor treatment by institutions in the past) for family members to question the value of therapy.

As therapists we may also be guilty of attitudes, beliefs, and practices that can get in the way of engagement. Such characteristics can include inflexible treatment hours (e.g., expecting working parents to join the therapy session but having our last appointment at 5 P.M.), therapy settings that are not welcoming, staffing and therapists who do not in any way share characteristics of our clients, and attitudes that might get in the way of fully embracing the input of the family. An example of the staff attitudes is worth expanding on. Research has shown that counselors often feel that family members cause too much conflict in therapy sessions, often verbally attacking and hurting the adolescent when they speak in therapy sessions (Baker et al., 1995). These are used as reasons why we should limit the involvement of "toxic" family members. The problem is that excluding these family members from the therapy session does not eliminate those painful and destructive processes at home. We believe this approach is ineffective because having the toxic communication and interactions occur in session allows the therapist to work on them, while keeping them out of the office just helps the behavior fester unchecked at home.

Therapists' Developing a Compelling Rationale for Full Family Involvement

By the time practitioners become family therapists, they have a firm belief that working with the entire family is a powerful way of helping an adolescent. Just keep in mind that the family you will treat did not attend those same classes and workshops that you did. It is a mistake to assume that the family will share the same perspective that all family members are needed in treatment. It is quite logical for a family member to think that only the person with the perceived problem (e.g., the adolescent displaying behavioral, substance use, and/or emotional problems) must change and therefore attend therapy. It becomes your job to give a rationale for family therapy that is convincing and compelling. In CIFFTA training and coaching, we train therapists to develop an *elevator sales pitch* that will truly give the family a new perspective on the problem and a family-level solution. The pitch can be unique to the therapist and one that fits best with their personality and approach. Examples of such sales pitches are "Even though things have not gone well, you are still an expert on your child, and I need your expertise to get therapy on the right track from the start"; "I am sure you have very specific values that you want to make sure your child learns and having you in sessions helps me make sure your child understands them"; or "You know best what has worked and what hasn't and hearing about this in session will help me be much more efficient in helping your child."

At times, in explaining the idea of family participation, the therapist may be able to lean on culture-related strengths of families. For example, Black and Latine family literature emphasizes terms such as *familism* and *familismo,* and *collectivism* as opposed to *individuality.* By citing this family orientation as a strength of the culture, the therapist can show how family therapy is consistent with that orientation of reliance on families in difficult times. An example might be "I know that you mentioned how important family is to you and I believe that by going through therapy as a family, you will be showing your daughter just how that works and how you are sticking with her through tough times. It is likely an experience she won't forget."

Another part of the therapist's task is to help the family see the problem and the solution within a systemic, interactional, and relational framework. Remember that we said that as a therapist, you must develop the systemic perspective, but the next step is to convey it to the family in a credible and jargon-free way. The family can begin to see that the problems occur within a meaningful relationship system (i.e., the family or larger contexts) and that all family members are impacted by and are impacting the presenting problem. Once they understand that they can impact the outcome just by talking to each other and connecting in a healthier way, they can feel a new sense of empowerment and hope. You might say:

> "Your daughter has a lot of resentment because of the immigration related separation you both experienced. If you can listen to her pain and the sense of loss she experienced when you left her, it will deepen your relationship and the bond you have. It will be hard for you to hear some of her anger and pain, and you may not agree with every part of her perspective, but if you can let her share these feelings, that experience will really change her heart and her behavior. I know one of your goals is for her to be more honest and open. We

can help her by having this conversation. Furthermore, if your new husband can be a part of it, he will also be part of the new bonding experience."

This is a critically important part of helping families understand how and why it is important to work with the entire family. Equally important, the adolescent must be helped to understand how and why the family needs to be involved in the treatment and how he or she can benefit from this type of treatment. Adolescents can also be reluctant to allow the family to participate in their therapy sessions. A therapist might say, "It sounds like your parents don't really get your perspective on some things. I would really like to help you, and I can do that by helping them take a fresh look at this issue."

The Cultural Worldview That Does Not Include Therapy

There are many culture-related beliefs and worldviews that do not endorse turning to the mental health system and therapy in difficult moments. For many Black, Latine, and other families there is a sense that private family matters should remain private, and one should not air dirty laundry in public. This is especially true if the family feels they have been treated unfairly by what they perceive to be a minority-unfriendly society or institution. It is also the case that in certain cultures there is a higher proportion of families that have a very traditional or hierarchical family organization. In these families, parents of an out-of-control and highly rebellious adolescent may feel particularly weak, defeated, and ashamed because they are unable to carry out their expected roles as effective leaders in the family. The disobedience of the adolescent can be experienced as a highly embarrassing failure of leadership and authority. In some ways, the introduction of the counselor amplifies the fact that the parents are unable to lead their family. The counselor must be particularly sensitive to the potentially threatening nature of their perceived role and attend to the family's hierarchical nature. The counselor can, from the very first contact, send the message that the parents are the leaders of the family even when things are not going well, and that the counselor cannot do the job of helping the youngster without their expertise and wisdom.

Hopelessness and Previous Failed Attempts at Change and Therapy

Therapists must be wary of labeling family members and caregivers as unmotivated, weak, and uncaring when what is underlying the actions and behaviors is pain and hopelessness. For many families, this is not the first therapy experience or efforts to help the child. The hopelessness currently in view can be directly proportional to the hope they felt at one time but that has been lost. Think of a parent of a child with self-harming behavior that has been to emergency rooms and tried other therapists. There are few things worse than knowing your child may harm or kill themselves and you are helpless to change that situation. Therapists must develop expertise at normalizing certain aspects of the help-seeking experience and instilling hope that things can get better.

What a CIFFTA Message to "Instill Hope" Sounds Like

- "It sounds like your family has gone through a lot in the past year! I think you are entering our program at just the right time and our services are designed for the very type of situation you are describing."
- "The stresses that you have described are related to being in a new culture and your daughter is struggling trying to figure out how to combine the old and new ways. Most new immigrant families go through this, and our counselors are trained to help you through this complex process. You don't have to struggle through this alone."
- "Your son is very lucky to have you still by his side after all that has happened and that is going to make all the difference for his future. You are to be commended for seeking services at this time."

Hope can be instilled when the clinician:

- Shows the links between the family's unique needs and what the program has to offer.
- Highlights that family members are doing some things well, even though the results are not yet what they expected.
- Conveys an understanding of what the family members are going through.
- Validates their concerns and stresses.
- Sheds light on individual and family strengths that are hidden (e.g., crises are opportunities to grow; worry comes from love and a need to protect).
- Normalizes the problem by showing it could be related to certain

stressors, including immigration, acculturation, discrimination, financial problems, and important changes within the family system.

Adolescents Who Are More Powerful Than Their Parents

When working with youth with severe behavior problems, it is not uncommon to run across adolescents who are powerful enough in the family systems that they can refuse to come to therapy. You can identify this situation when parents say that they waited for the adolescent to come home from school to ride together to the therapy session and the adolescents didn't come home. This is repeated several times and parents can't do much about it. Or the adolescent can outright refuse. *When adolescents have this much power, it is understandable that they do not want to enter a therapy that can increase the parents' power.* Most importantly, the adolescent can view the therapist as an ally of the parents and may be threatened by the prospect of facing such a powerful parent–therapist alliance. If the therapist allies only with the parents who are in a weakened position, the adolescent prepares themselves for one more power struggle and becomes entrenched in their refusal to enter therapy.

The best engagement approach when a therapist identifies a powerful adolescent is to reach out immediately to the youth to explore the adolescent's agenda and ensure that therapy works toward achieving their goals. The therapist must convey that the adolescent is seen as an individual who can make important decisions and bring about change (acceptance of power) rather than the person who can be forced to change. Both parents and therapists must convey to the youth that therapy will meet the adolescent's needs and agenda. For example, a therapist may say, "I think you are old enough to know what you want and need. I want to work with you so that you can get what you need and so that you are happy and successful. I imagine that having your parents on your back all the time is not something you are enjoying, and you have better things to do than battle them all the time. I think I can help them better understand your point of view and perspective."

An Adult Family Member Who Is Reluctant to Enter Treatment

In some instances, the person seeking treatment for the family (the initiator of the therapy) may tell the therapist that a family member is unlikely to want to come to treatment. At that key moment, one of the most important assessments that the therapist must make is whether the initiator of therapy seems to have an interest in keeping the other adult out of the therapy or whether they really want the other adult to attend treatment.

We will assume here that the initiator does not make excuses for why the other adult can't attend and that they make it clear that the other adult is needed and desired in treatment. There can be many reasons for the reluctance of the other family members, including having given up on the family or a desire to avoid a difficult and sensitive issue. Therapy may be feared as a vehicle that will place the adolescent issues on the back burner and focus on their own and/or couples' issues. For example, they may worry that the focus of treatment will become their couple's conflict, infidelity, or their substance use and aggressive behavior rather than the child's behavior. The therapist typically does not want to have multiple therapy sessions excluding an important caregiver because that may send the message that this caregiver is not needed or wanted. With each session that passes, the therapist may inadvertently strengthen a barrier between the disengaged caregiver and the therapy process or between the disengaged caregiver and the rest of the family. If too much time elapses, the disengaged partner may become convinced that the family members in treatment have already *poisoned the well* by placing them in a bad light.

The best route to take is to ask the family contact person's (who calls and initiates treatment) permission to contact the disengaged caregiver directly. During the call, the therapist needs to emphasize how much the person's perspective is needed, and to assure the reluctant caregiver that the therapy will focus on the adolescent's issues and not on global couples' issues. Therapists should not pressure the person to attend all therapy sessions. By asking the disengaged member to come to at least one or two sessions, the therapist then gains an opportunity for further engagement and joining. Keep in mind that the therapist must be prepared to take full advantage of the opportunity that one visit provides. You must give the reluctant family member an experience that really shows them why they are wanted and needed. If the therapist can show how their presence contributes to therapy success, future attendance becomes much more likely.

What a CIFFTA Engagement Contact Sounds Like

- "Thank you for your honesty, Ms. Robinson. Can you tell me if anyone else may be reluctant to participate in treatment? With your permission, I would love to contact them over the phone and ask for their help in getting our treat-

> ment of your daughter started right, even if they choose not to participate regularly. Is that OK with you?"
>
> - "Mr. Rodriguez, it would be very helpful to me to hear your perspectives on what is happening with your son and in your family. I can be much more helpful to your son if I understand your views on his behavior. Would you be willing to join us for at least one session and then you can decide whether to attend future sessions?"
>
> - "Ms. Jones [grandmother], it sounds like you have many caregiver tasks, and you know the family better than anyone. I cannot imagine being helpful without hearing your perspective."
>
> - "If you can come in for at least one session, I can hear your perspective and use your knowledge and expertise on the family to better help your granddaughter."

Initiator of Therapy Actively Keeping Another Caregiver Out of Therapy

In some instances, it becomes evident that the family member who is contacting the therapist rattles off a variety of reasons why the other caregiver cannot come to treatment and conveys that it is best to start with only certain family members. In this situation the caller is at best ambivalent and may be protecting the status quo by keeping certain family members out of therapy. Here the caller gives multiple justifications for why other family members cannot come to the therapy and quickly rejects therapist's suggestions on how the other family member can be included. Note that this is a very different situation from the one in which the initiator of treatment wants the other family members in treatment, but those other members are reluctant. And yet from a distance, these situations may look similar.

Why would an initiator of treatment want to keep a family member out? It may be that there is a possibility of a couple's conflict or infidelity that the initiator of treatment does not want to deal with in treatment. It may be that they do not want a grandparent or other extended family involved because that other parent-figure tends to be critical of the person's parenting. It may be that the other caregiver has a very different approach to handling the youth's problems (e.g., substance use) or perhaps doesn't even know about the substance use. There may be secrets or powerful issues that they want to keep hidden.

In this situation, it does not help to ask permission to call the other caregiver directly as you would do in the previous situation in which the initiator is not invested in keeping someone out of therapy. It would be a violation of the initiator's agenda. If you reach out to the other family member prematurely you may also lose the person who reached out to you. Instead, the therapist needs to detect this pattern early on and explore with the contact person the pros and cons of bringing in the other members. In effect, it is the contact person who must become motivated to have the entire family in session because they begin to see an advantage and benefit that outweighs their concerns. The therapist must ally with the initiator and open the door for expression of concerns of how therapy might proceed or take a wrong turn if the second caregiver joins the therapy session. The therapist can state that the initiator is overtaxed by taking on all the responsibility for change in the family and show the benefits of spreading the responsibility for change. The therapist must also ensure that the initiator's worst fears (e.g., being humiliated by the other family members) are not realized.

IDENTIFYING KEY FAMILY PROCESSES AND INTERACTIONS THAT NEED TO BE MODIFIED

While you are working on engagement and joining, another key competency is the identification of family process patterns. During engagement, you can begin to identify key family processes that can impact engagement and entry into therapy. This work continues when family members come to treatment. Once everyone is in the room, you can observe and "diagnose" the interactional and relationship patterns that characterize the family and their link to presenting problems. You will become skilled at *focusing on the family process and not on the content* of the story. If a family member is shouting at another family member and causing them to shut down, that is the most important indicator of what is happening in the family, much more important than the content or topic of the complaint (e.g., not taking out the garbage or not picking the kids up from school on time). The therapist can observe who shouts, at whom, how the target of the shouting responds (e.g., shutting down, shouting back, laughing, leaving the room), and how other family members react. Other family members may defend the target, support the person shouting, cry, or show that this interaction triggers the presenting symptom that brought the family to therapy (e.g., anxiety or explosive behavior). When the presenting symptom emerges in the middle of that sequence, the therapist may surmise that the presenting symptom may be a response to or have a role in stopping, the previous interaction that included the shouting and attacking.

Many therapists are trained to hear the story and follow the content of the story, and this can become a trap if they are distracted from seeing the interactional and relational processes that can be the most powerful maintainer of the problem. Fishman (2022) defines *process* as "the flow of interactions within a system. The observable transformations of members of a system *being* with one another" (p. 75). Problem processes often seen in family therapy (regardless of their content) can include (1) parental and caregiving figures who are expected to work together and support each other, but are undermining each other; (2) family members habitually jumping in, or being asked to enter the conversation, to defend or attack another while two people are having a productive dyadic conversation; and (3) someone shutting down or exploding when certain family members begin to disagree.

When you develop the skill of watching process carefully and not being distracted by content/topics, it will be easier to detect the repetitive interactions that get in the way of family well-being. Sometimes the therapist can use *tracking* to highlight an interaction and check in with the family regarding the observation. For example, a therapist may say, "It seems to me that when you start to disagree with your son, your wife comes in to help and diffuse the conflict, am I right on this? Does this happen often?" This statement doesn't seek to change the interaction or even judge it, but it highlights the pattern and asks the family to comment on the observation. It often brings the pattern into their awareness for the first time, or they might want to talk about why they do it. You will not need to learn their reason for doing it; it is helpful just showing how habitual and automatic it is. By checking in with them at the end (e.g., does that sound right or do you see this happening often), the observation becomes more of a collaborative exploration than any type of therapist pronouncement or interpretation.

GENERALIZING INFORMATION AND SKILLS

In Chapter 5, we described how individual sessions with the adolescent are used to generalize what is learned in psychoeducational sessions. In the same way, family therapy sessions are used to help the family with generalization of skills or knowledge. For example, the family can discuss what they learned about how depression manifests itself in family interactions and how it makes healthy interactions more challenging. Even though the discussion may be primarily about the youth, a depressed parent may realize they have more difficulty parenting just as a depressed adolescent may be more difficult to communicate with. The therapist can help family members have more meaningful, validating, and effective communication and interactions around the topic of depression and its impact on the family by exploring how it specifically plays out in *their* family. It is often the case that the thematic modules can normalize problems so that they do not seem so daunting, and they provide a language that allows more productive dialogue in the family.

In most families, we find it essential to provide the parenting module that focuses on the types of issues that often occur in the different developmental stages, how to support youth at the different stages, and how to set and communicate rules clearly and effectively. The parenting module also covers how to think about monitoring, reinforcement, and consequences at different ages. In the family sessions you can work to generalize what was learned in the psychoeducational sessions. Here the general strategies and recommendations are brought down to the family's real-life struggles and conflicts. What does it mean to be consistent when the two parents disagree on how strict to be and when one parent is much more permissive than the other? How does disagreement impact consistency and how can the parent-figures work to agree before addressing the youth? Conversations about parenting are an ongoing process in which therapists and families go back to discuss what was learned and how general concepts may need to be refined and tweaked so that they are more effective in the current situations and with the current crises.

At times, the modules may focus on adolescent skills, such as interpersonal skills. The module is delivered separately to the adolescent in an individually focused module session. Synergy between the therapy components is enhanced when the adolescent is encouraged to utilize the interpersonal skills in subsequent family therapy sessions. Here the therapist not only *coaches the adolescent* on how to use the skills most effectively but also *coaches the family on how to respond more adaptively* to the new adolescent behaviors. This latter work is important because families will often respond poorly to unfamiliar behaviors that are implemented in a less than artful way. Not surprisingly, when adolescents try new things (e.g., expressing their needs) for the first time, they are delivered in a way that sounds forced and even aggressive. In these instances, the therapist can help the family appreciate and validate the efforts the adolescent is making, and they can be coached on responding more adaptively.

> In the case of Maria, the separation between mother and daughter had contributed greatly to the emotional disconnection and distance between the mother and daughter. The Separations

psychoeducational module provided early on in therapy to the family helped to create a readiness for the family to process the separation, to share feelings related to the separation and to clarify misunderstandings in later family sessions.

The module normalizes the pain and sense of loss and resentment that often emerges in families during a separation. It helps move attention away from any family-specific animosity and instead, the feelings and difficulties are presented as common to many families who attempt to reunify after a long separation. The module work creates a "readiness" for more productive family sessions to work through the pain and sense of loss. In family sessions the work revolved around generalization of the lessons learned in the modules. Therapy focused on processing the pain and sense of abandonment while also modifying family interactions (e.g., defensiveness) that block the resolution of the issues. The therapist shaped conversations and enactments in which disclosure of pain was validated and heard without counterattacks.

REDUCING CONFLICTUAL AND HOSTILE INTERACTIONS

One of the most important competencies that the CIFFTA family therapist must learn is to effectively handle hostility and conflict. When working with multiple family members who are going through difficult times and who have been involved in disagreements and conflicts that they have been unable to handle, it is likely that the conflicts will erupt in sessions. The in-session hostility is merely an enactment of what occurs at home and by changing these enactments in the therapy room and *in vivo*, the family can take the new skills back home. To a certain extent, it is important for the therapist to allow some negativity to emerge in the early sessions so that they can identify the habitual and repetitive ways in which family members hurt, invalidate, criticize, and shut down other family members. The solicitation of an *enactment* in which the therapist elicits the habitual *family dance* (Minuchin & Fishman, 1981) reveals the areas that must be changed to create healthier relationships and is critically important to get to understand the family.

Enactments

An *enactment* occurs when family members interact among themselves as if the therapist were not present. The therapist remains very decentralized and on the periphery on purpose, so that the family can show its habitual way of relating to each other. The therapist watches family members discuss the issues and problems that they struggle with daily and sees firsthand *how* they handle the issues, treat each other, and communicate. The therapist can identify the adaptive and maladaptive ways of relating that they will want to enhance or modify.

Enactments may be *spontaneous* in which family members begin talking to each other naturally and without prompting. Enactments may also be *directed* in which the therapists ask the family to speak about an issue so that the patterns of relating become obvious. Later we will talk about a specific type of directed enactment in which the therapist introduces more adaptive ways of relating and asks the family to incorporate new messages into their interactions (e.g., shaping the interactions to be more positive and supportive).

On the other hand, the therapist cannot let the negativity and conflict escalate and go on too long. If the negativity is allowed to emerge and is then mishandled, it does not bode well for future family sessions. If negativity goes on too long, the family members may feel that therapy does not offer anything different and that the interactions are not changeable. The most vulnerable members will be particularly distressed that the therapist allowed the hurtful interactions to continue, and family members may feel they were embarrassed or humiliated in public. All these reactions to unbridled negativity and hostility are likely to cause the family to become more hopeless and less likely to return to the next session. The therapist must feel confident they have the strategies and tools that can stop the negativity when it is time to do so. Two powerful tools that the therapists have in the toolbox to gain control over negative interactions are blocking and reframing.

Blocking

A therapist who carefully watches the process and interaction patterns must be comfortable with being directive and capable of blocking or stopping certain communications that are unproductive and maladaptive. Much as you would see a traffic cop stopping certain cars to allow others to pass in a more controlled fashion, as a therapist you will need to stop certain communications that are overly negative or that are derailing important negotiations. Therapists that are not used to being this active in sessions will struggle at first with how to do this is a way that does not turn off the client or seem disrespectful. When the therapist is unskilled at blocking, they may also sound angry or controlling. It is important that therapists develop *and practice* ways of blocking that fit with their style (e.g., using humor) and that allows the blocking to occur without eliciting a negative response from the person who is blocked. Saying "I think you need to stop jumping in and interfering so the two of them can work this out" is much less effective than saying "What do you think of joining me as we sit back a bit and let's see how the two of them work this out?" Or "Mom, you work overtime to help your husband and son reach a resolution, what would you say to the idea of you and me letting them do the work today?" Or one can say, "That is a very important point you just made. Please hold on to it for a minute so that the two of them can complete the important work they started and then we can come back to give your point the time it needs." Practice makes the therapist more comfortable with the blocking intervention and less likely to come across as pushy or critical. Checking in with the client to see if it is okay also makes the blocking and redirection more collaborative. By developing effective and respectful ways of blocking, the therapist can take control of interactions and shape them into ones that are more adaptive, effective, and supportive of the changes the family would like to make.

Reframing

A considerable amount of clinical and research work has revolved around the important tool known as *reframing* (Minuchin & Fishman, 1981; Robbins et al., 1996). Reframing is a way to weaken negative attributions and begin to add complexity to the explanation of why things happen the way they do. When families begin therapy, they bring their own "frame" about the situation (i.e., their own explanation about why things happen and how). The frame or explanation is typically much more narrow, black and white, and simple than the reality. It also tends to leave out the love and desire to protect that are behind many behaviors. An important goal of family therapy is to help family members experience each other differently. To become open to a more complex, nuanced, and multifaceted explanation as to why things are happening the way they are.

In the middle of a highly negative and blaming interaction, reframing can introduce the deeper connections, hopes, aspirations, and positive intentions that family members have. The job of the therapist is to validate key aspects of the family's frame, while also expanding it and presenting a new more complex or positive one. This allows family members to perceive one another differently, in a more positive way that gives rise to the motivation to connect and understand each other in a healthier way. For example, when a youngster accuses the mother of constantly nagging and controlling, a therapist may say, "It sounds like your mother cares a lot about you and refuses to give up on you, although the caring and concern sometimes feels like nagging to you." A high-level reframe adds the positive and caring dimension but also acknowledges the complaint from the other family member. If the therapist only says, "Your mother cares about you and that is why she does that," the adolescent may feel invalidated and not heard and the therapist would be perceived as taking the mother's side in the argument. Acknowledging the youth's frustration alongside the mother's caring is key. A parent's close monitoring can be explained as love, concern, and protection, rather than as any special need or long-held desire to be controlling. Likewise, an adolescent's high level of emotion and intensity can be labeled as passion, which can be used positively and creatively in the future although it is sometimes more challenging to hear and respond to. For example, the therapist may say, "Mom, you have raised a strong daughter who will really be able to stand up for herself but sometimes her assertiveness may come across to you as a bit disrespectful." By including positive aspects and/or deeper connections and feelings, the therapist helps family members go beyond their habitual confrontational behaviors and become more vulnerable in their relationship. Words like *anger* or *fed up* are replaced by words like *pain, despair, desperation,* or *hurt*. Once the deeper family connections resurface, family members become more willing to *fight together* for the survival of the relationship and the family.

Changing the Interaction Sequence

So, we now know that you can use observation of enactments and tracking to identify the most habitual interaction patterns in the family that may lead to anger, hostility, and conflict. Identification of the triggers to conflict and the reinforcers are key. As you seek to change these interactions, we also know that blocking and reframing are effective tools. In the effort to change habitual interaction patterns there are additional concepts that are highly useful: circularity and complementarity. Although we did not name these concepts earlier, we did touch on their effects when we discussed the coercive process identified by Patterson and the way one can go about changing the pattern that surrounds the behavior (e.g., the reinforcing reactions). Because the individual is always seen in the context of their interactions and relationships to other people, we must constantly look at the way that the individual behaviors elicit the behaviors of others in the environment and the way the behaviors of others elicit, reinforce, or constrain the behavior of the individual. When behaviors complement each other and begin to fit together like a puzzle (e.g., someone is messy in an apartment, and someone loves to pick up) they become more and more predictable and rigid. There is a constant interplay of circular effects surrounding any behavior in question. This is more than just an interesting theoretical point; the identification of circular effects gives the therapist more treatment options. When seeking to change hostile and conflictual interaction patterns, one can seek to change any number of triggers or precursors that elicit behaviors and/or behaviors that reinforce the habitual pattern. Any change in the sequence opens a space for new and more adaptive behaviors to emerge. The therapist becomes even more aware that individuals tend to have more range of behavioral options in their repertoire than they tend to show in any given relationship (for a powerful and enlightening presentation of the related concept of *holons*, see Minuchin & Fishman, 1981). A submissive person at home may be assertive at work because that assertiveness is reinforced in that context. It helps the therapist to know that assertiveness is in the repertoire but constrained in the home environment. Because relationships that become rigid tend to constrain the behavioral options of the individual, any changes in the relationship context opens new possibilities. When a family member that is used to seeing anger in a spouse or family member (and reacting with even more anger or withdrawal) sees hurt and pain instead, that opens the door for a new set of reactions. The following box shows what this might look like in a therapy session.

Transcript from a Session on Substance Use Slips and Family Relationships

FATHER: (*in an angry and harsh tone*) John has continued to take drugs and I am ready to just give up on him. (*looking at son*) You are on your own from now on. I can't trust you or anything you say. Get into whatever trouble you want. I don't have the strength to keep fighting for you.

SON: (*in an angry tone*) You are finally being honest. You just want to give up on me. You don't love me as much as you always say you do. Fine, I will just go back to doing my thing.

THERAPIST: (*to the son*) It sounds like it meant a lot to you that your dad kept fighting and you still want him by your side.

SON: Yes, but he is angry at me, so he just drops me and doesn't care what happens to me.

> THERAPIST: What I have heard over our sessions is hurt and helplessness more than anger. When you love someone and can't save them from life difficulties, it is a painful feeling, isn't it Dad?
>
> FATHER: (*in a softer tone*) Of course, he knows that. It is not that I WANT to give up on him. It is just painful to look into the future and see what might happen to him.
>
> THERAPIST: (*to the father*) Sometimes John needs to hear it because that message gets lost in the struggle. It is actually a hopeful sign that a father wants to continue to help a son and that a son wants his father by his side. It is just that slips and relapses undermine hope. Sometimes the more hopeful we become, the more painful a slip is.
>
> THERAPIST: (*to both the father and son*) Does it make you feel sort of hopeless and helpless that some of these behaviors don't change so easily and that it is easy to slip?
>
> SON: Yes, it really is. Honestly, sometimes I just want to give up on myself.
>
> FATHER: I have never heard you say that.
>
> THERAPIST: Let's talk about how we can get back on track and how your support of each other can help the progress continue. Don't let the helplessness cause you to lose sight of what has been accomplished and how you have worked together.

SHAPING MORE ADAPTIVE AND SUPPORTIVE RELATIONSHIP INTERACTIONS

As you work to reduce negativity and hostility, you also work to open up and shape relationships and interactions to include more supportive, caring, and protective elements. Just as reframing allows those positive elements to be introduced, the shaping of family interactions ensures that these positive behaviors become part of the family's repertoire of behaviors. When conflict has been the most prominent aspect of relationships, it feels risky to let the guard down, express pain, and to show vulnerability and love again. It takes sustained work to make caring interactions habitual.

Family therapists identify and detect loving and caring communications even when they are very subtle and masked by conflict. The therapist highlights positive communications to change the way family members experience each other. A therapist might say, "Let me stop for a second because in the middle of everything, I heard your father say that your happiness and health is the most important thing to him. Did you always know that he felt that way? Do you hear it often?" Therapists also direct enactments that facilitate positive communications so that they become part of the repertoire that can be generated easily. For example, "Dad, your son says that he does not hear that very often and doesn't really know if he believes it. Can you say a bit more about how his health and happiness are so important to you—because after all, what else can be more important than this?" Often the father may look at the therapist and say that he really cares about his son. The therapist will say, "Dad, tell your son this directly. Turn toward him a bit and say it directly to him." By requesting this direct dyadic communication, the message has more intensity and meaning, and father practices his ability to say these types of things directly to his son. This will make it easier for similar communications to take place at home when the therapist is not there to act as a traffic cop. It is easy to lose the habit of generating loving statements when conflict has become chronic. Therapists can shape enactments that help make them easier to generate. Shaping communications, whether reducing conflict, or increasing support, validation, and caring communications is the most powerful tool the therapist has, and it fully takes advantage of the fact that the interactions to be modified are laid at the feet of the therapist *in vivo*. A therapist should never say, "now the two of you can try to speak directly at home as a homework assignment," unless the interaction was already completed successfully in the therapy room. Giving tasks to be completed at home without ever making them happen in the therapy room is typically a recipe for failure and frustration.

One task that the family has and that the CIFFTA therapists works to strengthen is the family's ability to buffer the youth and other family members from external stressors including things like discrimination, racism, and risky neighborhoods. The therapist works to make these environmental and societal pressures and stressors more visible and together they acknowledge how they are making their lives more difficult than they should be. It becomes very powerful when the therapist can help family members to validate the stress the youth face out in the world, and how that stress can push the youth to be less effective. It can become very meaningful when older family members can share their experiences and strategies that have worked for them in the past. When families can work on strategies together and support one another in the face of these powerful stressors, the family can buffer and protect the youth from the adverse effects that can otherwise result.

When working on supportive and caring communications in families, therapists must keep in mind that loving and caring relationships and communications look very different from one family to another and in different cultures. In some families and cultures, you may never see the highly affectionate family relationships you see in others. And yet, even the more understated and restrained ways of expressing love and affection can be extremely powerful when they are reintroduced or helped to resurface in the family. Therapists cannot force communications that don't fit the family culture, and they must be attentive to hear more subtle forms that are more natural to the family.

Another way in which culture interacts with supportive interactions revolves around the *acculturation gaps or discrepancies* we discussed in Chapter 2. It is often the case that as youth and their parents base their behaviors on different and seemingly competing worldviews, it becomes more difficult for the family to function as effectively as it is capable of. The natural tendency of younger family members to acculturate more quickly (often to a more individualistic or less family-oriented worldview) can be perceived by the parents and less acculturated family members as a rejection of the culture of origin and the values that the family holds dear. Following the introduction of the acculturation module that normalizes the varied worldviews shared within the family as part of well-established and predictable acculturation processes, the family therapy sessions can begin to expand the perspective of the family to include a more bicultural approach. This work includes open and caring conversations in which the powerful values of the culture of origin can be discussed and learned without having them imposed on the adolescent and without attacking the adolescent for having incorporated slightly different perspectives. For example, a therapist might say, "It is understandable that you want your daughter to understand the importance you place on family, it is one of the reasons you have never given up on her and are willing to come to every therapy session. The interesting thing is that the main culture of the United States places a lot of emphasis on the individual, assertiveness, and personal striving. Your daughter is growing up here, so it is also understandable that she is incorporating these values. We all incorporate the values around us. What will be key for your family is the ability to take the best of each of those perspectives and use them to be even stronger, rather than have the two perspectives battle each other. People who can maneuver both cultures and both sets of values tend to be particularly successful. Having both sets of values in your toolbox is almost like speaking two languages and you know how helpful that is."

WORKING WITH THE FAMILIES OF LGBTQ+ YOUTH

As we presented in Chapter 5, we have incorporated many advances related to work with LGBTQ+ youth and their families into CIFFTA. Sometimes families are very accepting and affirming of the youth's sexual orientation and gender identity. When they are not, the rejection can be very powerful and contribute to the high-risk profiles that many LGBTQ+ youth show. Therapist should keep in mind that the family's initial inability to accept and affirm the sexual orientation or gender identity endorsed by the child should not be cause for deciding that the family should be circumvented, and that further family work would be futile. In fact, there is a considerable paradigm shift that emphasizes the power of family acceptance of the youth and the importance of developing services that can help the entire family system through this transition (Ryan, 2010). Indeed, the family will be an important context and potential source of support long after the therapist is gone, and whenever possible it is well worth the effort to help create a more affirming, supportive, and validating environment (SAMHSA, 2014). The engagement of family members to work on issues they cannot easily accept is complex and the expectation should be that this requires careful and well-thought-out engagement work (Santisteban & Szapocznik, 1994; Santisteban et al., 1996). When we add cultural and worldview layers (e.g., acceptance being even more difficult and "out of the norm" within certain cultures) we can see the importance of therapists being well-prepared for the work. When therapists give up on the family prematurely or don't see the impact of cultural processes, they are not serving the adolescent well.

Acceptance of unexpected gender identities may be even more difficult for families to accept than sexual orientation. With increased visibility and access to information on transgender individuals in our society, young people have come out and or questioned their gender identity at early ages. This fact has made the family process of acceptance even more complicated because parents may question more and more whether the youth is equipped to make these complex decisions at an early age. The Family Acceptance Project (Ryan, 2010) has conducted groundbreaking work in this area and has shown that LGBTQ+ youth who report high levels of family rejection are 8.4 times more likely to have attempted suicide, 5.9 times more likely to report high levels of depression, and 3.4 times more likely to have used illicit drugs. Because these are the documented consequences and sequelae to minority stress (both inside and outside the home), we have developed CIFFTA treatment components (Mena et al., 2024a) that can help families in this area of work.

Therapists will often confront situations in which people, systems, and processes that are typically considered protective factors cease to be supportive and may become stressors. For example, when working with diverse families we note the high endorsement of religiosity and faith among Latine and Black families. These families may often lean on extended family and even the church family for social support in difficult times. These are typically described as important protective and resiliency factors. However, when an LGBTQ+ youth discloses their sexual orientation or gender identity to the parents, many parents report feeling that the extended family and church family will not be supportive. These contexts can also make acceptance of an LGBTQ+ identity more difficult and initial family rejection more likely (Hailey et al., 2020). Indeed, it may result in additional stress to the family situation because parents may feel the need to keep the information hidden. The parents may feel particularly alone and "in hiding" in a way that they are not used to, fearing that their typically supportive relationships will turn out to be unsupportive around this specific circumstance. In many ways the caregivers and family members begin to fear rejection in the same way that the youth does. Helping the family to maneuver through these uncharted waters can be a major support to the family. The therapist must be attuned to this possibility because the family may not naturally perceive or be aware of this change in their support system. CIFFTA has the components and strategies to help enhance the family's ability to buffer their youth from outside stressors and to help the family increase its affirmation of the youth.

Another complex family dynamic is when the youth has disclosed to only some family members and not others. Keeping important secrets in the family is typically avoided in family systems work because of the damage it can do to trust and communication. On the other hand, youth are often quite accurate in their assessments of who will be supportive and who will respond with a very painful rejection. The juggling of these processes must be done with great care. Therapists must be careful not to strongly encourage premature disclosure by the youth, under the assumption that it will always have a positive therapeutic outcome. It is also important not to villainize the family member who is taking longer to express acceptance. They need to be given time to process all the feelings they have (e.g., regret, concern, and culture-related factors that have been internalized) and to talk through the process. It sometimes helps adolescents to think through how long it has taken them to sort out their feelings while on their own journey. This sometimes helps them to grant their family members a bit more time for processing the changes.

In enhancing the material used in CIFFTA to address these issues, we collaborated with experts that specialize in working with sexual and gender minority youth, their caregivers, and the community. The enhancements include the real-life stories of young adults and family members who had gone through the coming-out process with differing levels of ease/difficulty. On video, parents shared why having their kids come out was difficult for them at the start and how they came to realize the importance of supporting and loving their children. We use video vignettes to present information (in English and Spanish) via three modules titled: "Coming Out, Finding Out," "Stigma and Mental Health," and "Support and Empowerment." These vignettes provide a vehicle for youth and families to hear that they are not alone in this process and that others experience similar situations. Furthermore, the videos help create a "readiness" in both youth and family members to address their concerns with open minds and open hearts.

WORKING WITH KEY SUBSYSTEMS AND FAMILY LIFE CYCLE STAGES

To facilitate the therapist's work to bring competence, success, and effectiveness to family interactions, it is helpful to have a roadmap for what success should look like. An important contribution by Minuchin and Fishman (1981) and colleagues, is the outlining of how subsystems work when they function adaptively. For example, the *couple subsystem* is composed of adults in a loving and caring relationship and designed so that they will support each other. They negotiate boundaries with extended family members, kids, and peers so that their couple relationships are private and protected. When emotionally difficult times emerge, the partner is expected to be empathic and supportive. As the therapist assesses the functioning of the family, a key question is whether there is a well-functioning and supportive couple subsystem.

When children are born, an entirely new set of demands are added to the members of the couple. The *parental subsystem* involves the work of being caregivers and this system sometimes adds new members such as grandparents who have caregiving roles. The blueprint for what behaviors should be present in the parental subsystem is often laid out in parenting skills and parenting practices manuals and include setting rules together, consistency, communication, rewards, and punishments. The couple subsystem and the parent subsystem include two very distinct sets of behaviors. An individual can be effective and supportive partners and yet be a very ineffective parent. The roles are quite distinct. It is like expecting an individual to be a good basketball player because they are a good tennis player. The skills and techniques needed may be very different even though being a good athlete helps. Typically, one of the things that is needed is good communication and agreement about things such as what parenting looks like and how much behavior control and monitoring will take place. The parenting subsystem can expand to include a grandmother, or an aunt, or a grandfather who take on significant caregiving roles. Sometimes it may even include older children who take on parenting functions. One of the keys to the parental subsystem is whether there is *agreement* on who does what and whether subsystem members support each other as opposed to undermining each other's parenting authority.

An important part of family therapy work is helping the parent figures to develop a better understanding of the adolescent's vulnerability and the long-term nature of the struggle that both the adolescent and the parents may have to deal with. Because of the behavior problems displayed by adolescents (e.g., delinquent behavior or substance use), it is often difficult for parents to look beyond the crisis behaviors to see the pain and struggles that the adolescent is experiencing below the surface. The CIFFTA therapist must help parents look beyond these acting-out behaviors and recognize the vulnerabilities and difficulties the adolescent is experiencing. Therapists must help parents understand the ways in which depression, anxiety, conduct problems, and ADHD manifest themselves, interact with each other, and impact the adolescent's behavior.

Finally, an often-overlooked subsystem is the *sibling subsystem*. Because siblings share so much history with schools, neighborhoods, parenting history, immigration, and other similar experiences, they can be a powerful support for each other. Therapists should keep in mind that it is possible to move beyond competitive struggles or past injuries and relationship ruptures and to recreate the support and bond that once existed or that can emerge for the first time. A mature and supportive sibling relationship can be a truly powerful context of support for any client.

Staying on Track

As in all of your CIFFTA work, ensure that the components are working in a synergistic fashion to meet both adolescent and family goals. The CIFFTA Treatment Plan and the CIFFTA Postsession Therapist Self-Report of Adherence are designed to help you stay on track as you plan family interventions and reflect on what was delivered in session. The following questions can help you keep track of how sessions go, which will help you keep the therapy focused and on track.

- "Did I engage all family members and join them around issues that are not 'problem'-related?"
- "If a reluctant member came in, did I make sure to involve that person in the session in a way that they experienced how important their participation is?"
- "Did I make the family feel comfortable with the idea of therapy and ensure I am not seen as an adversary or ally of the system?"
- "Do I understand the environmental stressors the family must live with and help them acknowledge and understand how to minimize the harmful effects?"
- "Do I have a good sense of the effectiveness of parenting in the different parenting domains and help them become more effective in the areas they struggle with most?"
- "Did I identify knowledge gaps that I can help the family to fill, and did I provide the needed modules?"
- "Do I have a good understanding of the family environment and help them improve the quality of the relationships, increase support, and reduce conflict?"
- "Did I use the family sessions as the arena in which to shape and reinforce more adaptive family relationship patterns and generalize skills learned?"

SUMMARY

In this chapter we have shared perspectives, strategies, innovations, and specific techniques for addressing many of the most pressing challenges that emerge when working with families around different presenting issues. We covered competencies like developing a systemic conceptualization and engaging reluctant family members, to techniques used to reshape negative and harmful family interactions and enhance protective interactions. We described in some detail specific ways of working when acculturation and/or contextual stressors are present and some of the unique issues in working with families of LGBTQ+ youth. We ended the chapter sharing a perspective on how to enhance the adaptive nature of interactions within family subsystems and in different life cycle stages.

7

CIFFTA's Psychoeducational and Modular Component

This chapter focuses on CIFFTA's psychoeducational modules, procedures for using them, and solutions to implementation challenges that can arise. You can utilize CIFFTA's modules to provide structured and systematic presentations of information on specific topics that are uniquely relevant to each of your youth and families. (Please follow this link to the CIFFTA online training platform: *www.guilford.com/santisteban-materials*.) When attempting to bring about behavior change, it is often helpful for clients to have foundational knowledge of specific topics and issues at the core of the presenting problem. This includes normalizing the problems and helping families understand that many families go through similar issues and overcome them. The foundation provided by the psychoeducational modules facilitates the behavioral changes sought by the CIFFTA individual and family therapy sessions. Information delivered via psychoeducational modules provides context and creates a frame for the difficulties the youth and/or family are facing. The goal is to increase the youth and family's *readiness* to incorporate more adaptive ways of functioning and to improve family communication and connection. It is helpful when you can convey that the youth and family have expertise regarding their situation, and that your role is to collaborate with them in ways that they determine would be most helpful to them. If the youth and/or family sense that you are judging them or lecturing them with information because the family members are deficient in a certain area, they may disengage and discontinue services.

At its core, CIFFTA seeks to (1) facilitate youth and family movement toward flexibility and behaviors that are increasingly adaptive, (2) increase the youth's use of effective skills and goal setting, and (3) increase the family's ability to support, guide, accept, care for, and love the youth. The modification of barriers that impede progress can include (1) the reduction of conflict and the repair of relationship ruptures that interfere with smooth family functioning and support; (2) the identification of acculturation- and immigration-related experiences and systemic/structural stressors that contribute to conflict in relationships; (3) providing information or skills needed for effective family and youth functioning; (4) identifying issues that interfere with parental acceptance of the youth; and (5) identification and modification of adolescent snares (Moffitt & Caspi, 2001)—such as substance use, emotion dysregulation, and deviant peers—that can block healthy youth development and functioning. CIFFTA's psychoeducational component directly supports these goals and addresses the barriers via education and information.

Psychoeducational modules are delivered in separate didactic sessions because regular family and individual therapy sessions do not always facilitate the family's learning of important facts relevant to the youth and family (e.g., drug effect education, triggers and motivations for self-harm, processes of acculturation, and parenting practices). CIFFTA's psychoeducational component provides parents and adolescents with focused information and educational sessions on specific areas that are relevant to the family. Material uses terminology that caregivers and adolescents can digest. Unlike the work in family therapy, here content is emphasized more than process. This format facilitates the delivery of the content without being sidetracked by other issues that are the focus of regular therapy sessions. When needed therapists can redirect the youth and/or family to stay focused on the content while reassuring them that they will be delving deeper into the therapeutic work in the next family or individual therapy session. Family process issues such as how the family works together in addressing a content area and how the module content can be applied to their family are flagged in the module sessions and then become a focus of the next therapy session. This work carried over from a module session to a therapy session is called *module generalization* in the CIFFTA model (see the section "Generalizing the CIFFTA Module" later in the chapter). While it may be tempting to use the psychoeducational modules as a stand-alone intervention, we feel that they only have their maximum effect when fully integrated into a larger therapy model. Without the focused generalization work that identifies and modifies all the maladaptive behaviors that constrain change, it is unlikely that psychoeducation can have a lasting effect.

MODULES FOCUSED ON YOUTH SYMPTOMATOLOGY

In this section we present brief descriptions of the modules that we have developed for the CIFFTA psychoeducational component. The selection of modules allows for flexibility to add content that is highly relevant to the specific youth and family you are working with. For example, we developed modules on self-harm and issues specific to LGBTQ+ youth and their families that might also be contributing to higher rates of self-harm in these youth. We also developed a module on social media to address the increasing risks related to social media use in youth. Versions available for parents also help them understand the pros and cons of social media and prepare them to provide more effective guidance and leadership on these issues.

Depression Module

This module helps youth and families understand the complex feelings and behaviors that surround depression. Symptoms of depression are sometimes hard to detect in adolescents because they involve internal feelings they may not understand or openly discuss, and because they can be masked by acting-out behaviors such as substance use and antisocial behavior. The module helps family members identify key warning signs that adolescents may be going through a period of depression. After recognizing that there is a problem with depression, families can be instrumental in supporting adolescents and helping them find effective coping strategies. The Depression module helps the adolescent and family better understand and identify symptoms and characteristics of depression, strategies that may help the youth cope, improve communication about the topic, and consider treatment strategies including the role of medication in the treatment of depression. When family members become more knowledgeable about the symptoms, they can more readily support the youth and validate their experiences.

Attention-Deficit/Hyperactivity Disorder Module

The ADHD module provides information about the symptoms and characteristics of ADHD, ways in which they show up in the youth's daily life, strategies that caregivers and youth can implement to help the youth manage, and treatment strategies including the role of medication in the treatment of ADHD. It helps the youth and family think more specifically about the types of changes that can be made to the home environment and schoolwork strategies that can help alleviate the symptoms. Many minoritized families are concerned that their youth may be diagnosed and labeled prematurely and even overmedicated. We use the module to open the door to a respectful dialogue about this and any other concerns they have.

Self-Harm and Suicide Risk Module

This module focuses on facilitating a greater understanding of the intimidating nature of self-harm. It is easy for family members to minimize or deny the problem as a way of coping with something that is so threatening and painful to acknowledge. The module serves to reduce stigma and shame related to self-harm. It presents the overall rates of self-harm and suicide ideation, the distinction between the motivations for nonsuicidal self-injury versus suicide-related behavior, and the intrapersonal and interpersonal triggers to self-harm and suicide behavior. Intrapersonal (inside the person) reasons might make teens vulnerable to self-harm behavior, and interpersonal (between people/outside in the world) reasons might be the triggers leading to self-harm. Self-harm is defined in the module as a behavior that is intentionally inflicted (it is done on purpose) and has immediate physical consequences (the body is hurt and damaged in some way). The damage can vary from mild scratches to deadly/lethal injuries. Injurious behavior that starts out less severe can become increasingly severe over time. Warning signs shared with youth and caregivers include thinking or talking about self-injury, talking or thinking about death, expressing that life is not worth living or that there is no reason to live, making comments or jokes about committing suicide, increased isolation or alone time, and avoiding social activities. The module also discusses the ways to treat self-harm and prevent suicide along with interventions that can normalize the helplessness, hopelessness, and shame that family members often experience.

Health Promotion Module

The goal of the Health Promotion module is to provide information to caregivers and adolescents about how to live a healthy lifestyle. Information about healthy eating healthy habits, fitness, sleep, experimentation with drugs, and the effects these have on the body and brain are shared. This is an excellent vehicle for discussion about alcohol, smoking, and other substance use before they are initiated, and, as such, serves the goal of prevention. The connection between mental health and physical health is also discussed. The act of promoting a healthy family conversation around these issues before it becomes necessary to confront a major problem is itself a prevention intervention.

Alcohol and Other Substance Use Module

This module discusses risks associated with alcohol and other substance use and reviews specific information about different classes of substances. It explains how substance abuse can be harmful to youth's development and provides caregivers with educational material about different ways of helping their youth if they are demonstrating substance misuse problems. The module helps youth and caregivers to understand that there can be hidden mental health issues such as anxiety or depression underlying the substance use and that even if the substance use is stopped, one must still address the underlying conditions to avoid relapse. Substance use can often mask more internalizing behaviors. It is also important for youth and family members to know that substance use can potentiate other major problems such as self-harm, suicide, and violence toward others. Indeed, many of these other problem symptoms can be alleviated by reducing substance use. Separate modules for youth and for caregivers are available. Having separate sessions is often helpful because both caregivers and youth can be more honest about use patterns (e.g., which peers promote use or use before school) and their lack of knowledge of some aspects of drug effects. This can set the stage for more productive family sessions.

Risky Sexual Behavior Module

The literature shows that youth who misuse substances and display other risky behaviors are at risk for HIV and STIs because of their risky sexual behaviors. This module teaches about sexual behaviors, safer sex practices, STIs, and pregnancy prevention. It also covers the importance of caregivers talking with adolescents about sexually risky behaviors and provides information for how caregivers can engage in these conversations with youth. Research has suggested that although parents can help their youth stay safer by having conversations about safe sex, at times parents feel they lack the information and terminology needed to guide their youth on this topic. The module for parents provides them with the information and confidence to lead discussions about this topic more effectively. Separate modules for youth and for caregivers are available.

Trauma Module

Many youth have experienced a traumatic event at some point in their lifetime. When working with immigrant youth, there can be additional traumatic experiences in the country of origin (often the reason they left everything and fled), others related to the process of crossing borders, and others related to having had family members deported. The impact and the severity of the trauma can vary greatly. This module defines trauma for youth and caregivers, normalizes exposure to trauma, explains the symptoms of posttraumatic stress disorder (PTSD), reinforces the notion that the trauma was not the youth's fault, and emphasizes that caregiver/family support can be powerful. Participants do not have to meet the full threshold for a PTSD diagnosis to benefit from this module. The goals of the Trauma module are (1) to provide psychoeducation for adolescents and their families on traumatic stress, and its prevalence and its effects on their thoughts, feelings, behavior, and body; (2) to discuss the long-term consequences that can occur if trauma is left untreated; (3) to discuss the effects of trauma on family functioning, and opportunities found within the family and their community to promote resilience; and (4) to help prepare families with cognitive and relaxation strategies. The module covers the following topics:

- What is trauma and PTSD?
- Prevalence of trauma and PTSD in youth
- Signs and symptoms of trauma
- Trauma reminders
- Trauma and the family
- The role of cognitions and emotions in the development of trauma symptoms and PTSD
- Introduction to the cognitive triangle
- Teaching family relaxation strategies
- Identifying the most distressing/impactful event
- Recognizing destructive/unhelpful communication patterns
- Increasing parental validation and improving skills to prevent escalations.

The module instills hope that treatment can help, and growth can occur following the trauma. Although CIFFTA cannot be considered a treatment specifically designed for trauma, much of the family work that we do (e.g., validation, support, open communication, and learning to listen to painful experiences without defensiveness) is highly recommended in trauma work. This module helps the therapist to be prepared to address the issues that sometimes emerge once treatment for other presenting problems has started. It also helps us to assess when a referral to a more intensive trauma treatment is needed.

GENDER IDENTITY AND SEXUAL ORIENTATION MODULE

As we discussed in Chapter 5, adolescents juggle myriad changes in the formative years and part of this work entails finding out who they are. This can include their identity regarding race, ethnicity, sexual development, sexual orientation, and gender identity. While belonging to the LGBTQ+ community can be a source of strength, it also brings unique challenges. It is important to recognize how sexual orientation and gender identity relates to mental health. In the case of LGBTQ+ youth, this time can be experienced with great anxiety, distress, and isolation as they discover their developing orientation and identity often in the context of marginalization and discrimination. The goal of the module is to incorporate basic education and training for therapists on mental health and well-being concerns related to rejection, discrimination, and stigma around gender and orientation stereotypes. This module prepares the therapist to have a respectful, supportive, affirming, and open discussion with the adolescent. When the caregivers are aware of the adolescent's thoughts and feelings about these issues, we also offer a module to the caregivers to help them process the information, and work toward acceptance rather than rejection of the youth. Helping loved ones to process this important information in a healthy way is important to the well-being of the youth and family. Of course, the work with families can only occur once the youth has disclosed to the family. The module covers the following topics:

- LGBTQ+: What's in a name?
- The CASS Identity Development Model, which describes six stages of identity development for LGBTQ+ youth
- Intersectionality: LGBTQ+ youth and families (Latine, Black and African American)
- Myths and stereotypes
- Health considerations for LGBTQ+ youth
- Risks associated with LGBTQ+ identities
- Protective factors
- An activity to demonstrate the power of perspectives
- Resources

SKILLS DEVELOPMENT MODULES

Among the challenges adolescents face is to figure out how to interact effectively in new more complex settings with school personnel, peers, health professionals, extended family, and even in a different way with parents. It is often the case that they are unprepared to process their needs, thoughts, and feelings. We have found that the modules developed by Marsha Linehan (2014a, 2014b, in press-a, in press-b) as part of her DBT work can be helpful if carefully integrated into a larger treatment model. We are grateful that we had the opportunity to work with Dr. Linehan, and her generosity fueled our efforts to integrate these aspects into CIFFTA.

Emotion Regulation Module

As any therapist knows, one of the presenting problems with adolescents is often emotion dysregulation, anger, and/or explosiveness. This can be particularly central to youth who self-harm or misuse substances. The emotion dysregulation is often the trigger to harmful behaviors. This module focuses on teaching adolescents three things: (1) how to identify their emotions and triggers; (2) how to reduce their emotional vulnerability; and (3) how to react to negative emotions in a way that is not impulsive and that leads to positive outcomes. The module defines emotions and emotion regulation and provides education on why it is helpful to regulate emotions and what happens when our emotions control us instead of us controlling our emotions. Skills such as ABC Please (Accumulation of Positive Experiences, Building Mastery, Coping Ahead, Treat Physical Illness, Balanced Eating, Avoid Mood-Altering Drugs, Balance Sleep, Get Exercise), opposite action, centering, and mindfulness of current emotion are covered in depth.

Interpersonal Effectiveness Skills Module

Another important aspect of adolescence is identifying and acknowledging their own needs and wants and figuring out effective ways of getting their needs met (Linehan, 2014a, 2014b, in press-a, in press-b). This module focuses on teaching adolescents three things: (1) how to be more effective at selecting and obtaining goals; (2) how to keep important relationships positive; and (3) how to develop and maintain self-respect and feel good about oneself. When we combine this with our family therapy sessions, we can directly shape, *in vivo*, the adolescent's use of these skills in family interactions and negotiations. Youth practice how to express needs, how to approach family members in the most effective way, and how to process the fact that not all needs and wants are satisfied. The social skills component also includes information on why friends are important and how to make friends who impact the adolescent positively. It teaches the youth about maintaining good friendships through the set of skills related to perspective taking. The module concludes with a discussion of what peer pressure is and how to manage harmful peer pressure.

Distress Tolerance Module

The Distress Tolerance module is designed to assist youth in responding to intense and negative emotional experiences. The goals of the distress tolerance skills are to help the adolescent: (1) tolerate difficult situations and emotional pain when the problem cannot be immediately solved, (2) survive a crisis without making it worse by acting on impulsive urges, and (3) bear pain skillfully by not engaging in problem behavior including substance use, self-harm, and eating disorders. Two types of distress tolerance skills are shared with the youth. The first type, Crisis Survival Skills, helps change our experience by pushing the painful situation out of mind temporarily. Distractions can help us get our minds off the thing that is causing us to feel intense painful emotions. Distraction using Wise Mind ACCEPTS skills is taught. The second type, Radical Acceptance skills, teaches us to fully accept painful experiences that cannot be changed. Strategies to assist in managing emotional and physical reactions to negative events are reviewed and the adolescent creates an individualized plan that they will implement when intense crisis events occur.

MODULES FOCUSED ON CULTURE AND CULTURE-RELATED STRESSORS

There are a number of immigration- and acculturation-related experiences that can directly impact youth and family well-being. CIFFTA includes a set of modules that you can use to help families identify, give meaning to, and better manage the types of stressors they frequently confront.

Acculturation Module

As presented in Chapter 2, acculturation is a complex and powerful process. It involves challenging and changing established beliefs, worldviews, values, and behaviors. Stress can emerge due to tensions during this transition process. When you widen the lens from the individual to also include entire families, you can see that additional stress can emerge when family members acculturate in different ways and at different rates.

Based on Berry's acculturation model (Berry & Sam, 1996) the module normalizes the process of acculturation and the process by which family members acculturate at different rates. Although the most common pattern was for adolescents to acculturate at a faster rate than their parents and older family members, we are now seeing youth who are not happy they were brought to the United States (or the way they are treated in the United States) and do not wish to acculturate at all. They prefer to keep their culture of origin and seek to return to their country of birth. The Acculturation module includes information on internal family processes and how they are influenced both positively and negatively by acculturation processes. Family processes that are impacted include socialization processes, parental leadership, parenting practices, bonding, communication, conflict resolution, worldview regarding individuation, and emotional and physical closeness. When this process can be normalized and families understand that adolescent acculturation is to be expected and healthy, there is less feeling that the adolescent is choosing to reject their culture of origin. The reduction of blame opens the door for family support and an honest discussion about the pros and cons of each set of cultural values and beliefs. It allows family members the opportunity to take the best of what each culture has to offer and consider the benefits of being bicultural.

Immigration-Related Separation Module

Also as discussed in Chapter 2, a common occurrence in immigrant families is the separation of youth and their caregivers during the immigration process. This occurs when a parent comes to the United States ahead of their children and reunites with them years later. The expectation that this will be a smooth and happy reunion does not consider that there is pain, a sense of loss, and many questions that must often be processed. The Immigration-Related Separation module facilitates the repair and rebuilding of the parent–adolescent relationship following an immigration-related separation. In broad terms, the module seeks to (1) increase the level of empathy of all family members regarding what they have all gone through; (2) allow each family member to express their pain and anger without accusations; (3) create a frame that conveys that the ability to listen to painful experiences creates stronger and deeper relationships (which is desired by the family members); (4) clarify misconceptions; (5) increase overall communication; and, perhaps most importantly, (6) decrease defensiveness so that 1–5 above are possible. The ability to process these life events facilitates the deepening of the adolescent–caregiver relationship.

Discrimination Module

This module can be helpful to the therapist when a youth and/or family report that they experience discrimination in their daily lives. The module defines discrimination, provides examples, and explains how this type of experience can negatively impact mental and physical health. It also emphasizes the possible impacts on relationships. The discussion questions allow family members to reflect on their experiences and share personal perspectives on the topic. Rather than allow individuals to have to deal with this on their own, we want therapists to think about its implications for families and to mobilize the family to support and guide each other in this difficult context. The CIFFTA therapist will want to use the family strengths and resources to buffer the youth from the negative impacts, and the module provides opportunities for parents to take a mentoring role on how to survive this chronic stressor.

MODULES FOCUSED ON DEVELOPMENTAL STAGE CHALLENGES

The adolescent developmental stage is complex and there are enormous challenges that the adolescent faces for the first time. CIFFTA includes a set of modules that seek to help the adolescent to appreciate the complexity of the situations they are facing and provide guidance on how to handle stressors in the most effective ways.

Teen Dating and Interpersonal Violence Module

Teenagers seeking treatment are often caught in unhealthy and dissatisfying relationships. It is helpful to have material that will facilitate a thoughtful discussion of this important process. The Teen Dating module includes information for adolescents on how to find a good partner and how to be a good partner. It also describes what respectful relationships look like, what controlling relationships look like, how they can deteriorate, and what teen dating violence looks like. The Relationship Attachment Model (RAM), which refers to the five bonding dynamics that create a feeling of attachment in a relationship (i.e., know, trust, rely, commit, sexual touch) is presented. The module also includes warning signs of dating violence, what to do if the youth or someone the youth knows is in trouble, and available resources.

Social Media Module

It has become increasingly evident that social media can accelerate and potentiate the good and the bad in an adolescent's life. Social media has been found to exacerbate the difficulties that a youth is experiencing. For example, it used to be that a youth could get away from school bullying by leaving the school and arriving at home. With social media, this is no longer the case. Bullying can occur 24/7 and can even be more powerful because of the permanence of videos and pictures. Topics covered include facts and positive aspects of social media and the internet, introduction to online safety, social media platforms, social media and mental health, social pressures, risky behaviors and safety, warning signs, legal issues related to social media, and supervision and parental controls. Separate modules for youth and caregivers are available.

MODULES FOCUSED ON PARENTING AND THE FAMILY

Because of the importance of effective parenting for any family with a child or teenager who is struggling, we offer a parenting module to all families in our programs. In addition, we have modules that can address the unique circumstances that often surround blended and single-parent families.

Parenting Module

We believe that all caregivers of youth seeking treatment can benefit from a conversation focused specifically on the challenges and opportunities that are part of parenting. Whether we are talking about parenting a youth with unique mental health needs, or parenting in risky and stressful neighborhoods and environments, or parenting in unique circumstances such as in separated couples, single-parent, or blended families, it is powerful to strengthen the parenting unit to support the family and youth. The Parenting module begins by discussing child development and appropriate milestones up to age 18. This helps parents to better understand unique behaviors their children may display and to prepare for changes in stages of development from childhood to early and later adolescence. Next, it addresses specific parenting techniques such as rewards, active ignoring, effective commands, monitoring, and limit setting. Not only do parents get the opportunity to evaluate what works and what doesn't work for them, but the module also provides parents with strategies that can make their parenting more effective. Part of this conversation focuses on how something as important as monitoring may look different depending on the age of the youth. We have also begun to emphasize validation more than ever, as we teach parents that they can be validating and support the youth having an opinion even when they disagree with that position or opinion. Healthy general communication, healthy attachment, and the importance of self-esteem in teenagers are also addressed. When there are multiple caregivers, the module emphasizes the importance of having caregivers communicate effectively and support each other. Culture and how it can impact parenting is a focus throughout the entire module.

Single Parenting Module

The Single Parenting module discusses stresses associated with being a single parent and strategies for managing the stress and challenges. It encourages a single parent to think about and discuss their specific stressors and coping strategies. The module also addresses unique aspects of single parenting for Latine families. Parenting is difficult enough when there are two involved parents, so when the responsibility of parenting is placed on only one parent the task becomes even more difficult. The module shares helpful information and validates the experiences of the parent. Single parents tend to experience high stress around not having enough time to spend with the children, juggling childcare, the finances, their personal needs, and having sole responsibility for childrearing. Single parents often find it difficult to achieve a balance between focusing on their own needs and the needs of others. When there is no balance or expectations are too high, the parent can become frustrated and overwhelmed. These feelings can lead a single parent to isolate or withdraw from people or activities that can serve as resources. Parents can also develop an unhealthy relationship with their children. A single parent may begin confiding in a child, directly or indirectly seeking emotional support and validation, and/or simple companionship that is not appropriate for the child's age. When a parent does this, it may inadvertently lead to a loss of authority that is needed to guide and discipline. Regardless of the source and type of stress, managing these pressures is important. For Latines, family unity is a priority and in searching for support or resources, they will often turn to family members including extended family and relatives. Assistance can range from helping with home repairs to child care issues to financial support. The module concludes with suggestions for ways a single parent can take care of themselves.

Blended Family Module

The processes and dynamics that come with forming a blended family are often underappreciated. Blended families often originate from loss, either a death or a divorce, which may be emotionally difficult for all involved. The Blended Family module addresses the transition to a new family environment and encourages the family to discuss their feelings about how relationships form and change. The module provides information to help understand the transition and normalizes difficulties that can arise when two families join to become one. There are several challenges to a new family composition, including development and maintenance of relationships:

- The couple is attempting to solidify their new relationship.
- Parents have preexisting relationships with their children that need enhancing.
- Relationships between the stepparent and the new spouse's children are beginning.
- Children of both adults may also be forming stepsibling relationships.

Important topics related to the new family, such as family structure, new roles, and how to develop strong relationships in the blended family are addressed.

Modules Focused on Family Advocacy in the Youth's Ecology

Parental advocacy in school, neighborhood, health system, and legal contexts is key to adolescent well-being. Yet many parents may lack the perspective, skills, or worldview that facilitates fulfillment of this role. It is easy to prematurely label parents as overly passive or detached when in fact they are intimidated and lack knowledge about the complex systems that their youth participate in. The therapist can help prepare caregivers for this work on behalf of the adolescent. This set of modules educates caregivers about the legal, school, and psychiatric systems and how to effectively navigate them. These systems are complex and navigating them can be further complicated by minority status, culture, and language barriers. Often, caregivers carry cultural values that say, "You do not question doctors or authority figures." Yet remaining silent or avoiding these systems can have serious negative consequences for youth. These modules help caregivers learn about the systems, why it is important to advocate for youth, address cultural norms related to interacting with these systems, and help caregivers gain confidence to address the systems and advocate for their youth.

Legal System Module

Navigating the legal system can be a daunting task, particularly for caregivers trying to understand the process their child goes through in the juvenile justice system. By helping caregivers to better understand the system, the roles of the different players (e.g., public defenders, case managers, probation officers) and how to intervene, we can help them assert their parental power in this legal domain. The module also provides details about offices within the system that specialize in immigration issues and that can assist families, especially when there is concern surrounding interacting with the law. Youth and caregivers are provided with information about the following topics:

- Current statistics related to juveniles in the legal system
- General information about the local juvenile services division
- The different players in the system and their roles (e.g., parole officer, public defender)
- The process when a youth is taken into custody
- What happens posttrial
- Helpful resources
- When a youth is being tried as an adult

School Module

The School module provides information that can facilitate caregivers' connection to the school system and offers important steps that can help them communicate more effectively with school administrators and teachers. Caregivers may feel overwhelmed by the school system and unsure how to become involved in their youth's school world. Staying connected to school is a key to ensuring a youth's success. Communication issues, cultural barriers. language difficulties, busy schedules, and academic or behavior issues are among the things that are addressed in the module to increase caregiver confidence to engage with their youth's school and to advocate for them with school administrators.

Medication Module

The Medication module is designed for youth and their caregivers who are being referred for a psychiatric evaluation or other referrals that may include a prescription for medication. The module addresses family concerns about medications and discusses the importance of medication compliance and medication adjustments that are often required. If family members are not prepared for the medication adjustments that are typically needed, they are likely to prematurely discontinue the medication without medical advice. Caregivers are empowered to question the costs and benefits of the medications as appropriate. The module encourages family members to discuss their feelings about medication and includes a list of questions that families can bring with them to the appointment to structure their session.

HOW TO IMPLEMENT CIFFTA'S PSYCHOEDUCATIONAL COMPONENT

The first step in implementing CIFFTA's psychoeducational component is to select the modules that are most relevant to the youth and the family. As discussed in detail in Chapter 4, data from the intake assessment, Tailoring Report, and the CIFFTA clinical interview are used to identify the modules that are most appropriate for each youth and their family. Depending on the profile for each family, certain modules will be indicated, and others can be deemed not necessary. For example, if youth depressive symptoms are high, the parent is a single parent, and acculturation stressors exist, then the Depression, Single Parenting, and Acculturation modules are relevant for the youth and family.

A youth/family's Tailoring Report may indicate that a high number of modules are relevant for them (more than five modules). This is especially true for cases that report high-risk behaviors and symptoms. The therapist and family together will need to prioritize an initial set of modules (three to four); otherwise, both the therapist and the youth/family can become overwhelmed. The decision of which modules to prioritize should be made collaboratively with the youth and with the family. It is recommended that the Parenting module be delivered to all CIFFTA families, and it should be delivered early in treatment because it will facilitate the parenting work throughout treatment.

Choosing the Family Members Who Will Receive the Modules

Certain modules are given to the parents alone, for example the Parenting module. Other modules are given to adolescents alone, for example, the Emotion Regulation module, the Interpersonal Effectiveness Skills module, and the Teen Dating and Interpersonal Violence module. There are also modules that are delivered to parents and adolescents together. Examples are the Health Promotion module, the Immigration-Related Separation module, the Depression module, and the Medication module. Finally, there are modules that both youth and caregivers can receive, however, the therapist may want to deliver them separately and then come together for module generalization. One example is the Risky Sexual Behavior module. This module is best delivered separately so that both youth and caregivers feel comfortable sharing information about behaviors and concerns that they may have. The same is true for the

Alcohol and Other Substance Use Module. Although eventually we want to have full discussions on these topics with all family members present, initially it is best to give them the safe space to be totally honest about their behaviors and their concerns.

Choosing When and How to Deliver the Module

The CIFFTA psychoeducational component should be integrated into the treatment after the engagement and joining phase and MI strategies have been implemented. When youth and families are open to the treatment process and motivated, they are better able to receive the modules. Modules are usually implemented at a rate of 1 every 2 weeks or so. To facilitate delivery to Latine families, the modules are available in English and Spanish, and some are available in the form of videos that can be viewed anywhere and at a time that is most convenient to the youth and family. Modules are typically delivered in one 60-minute session although some more complex modules such as Parenting and Interpersonal Effectiveness Skills can be delivered over two sessions. It is also possible that a new issue arises with the youth and/or family that requires the therapist to revisit the content of a module that was already delivered. For example, a youth may need to go back to the Emotion Regulation module if emotional outbursts continue well after the module has been delivered and module generalization is not having the desired impact. Or a therapist may need to review the Parenting module again with caregivers if a new issue arises that causes a breakdown in the parenting subsystem. Going back to the content of a module can be effective as it allows the family to work through how they can apply the content to new and different situations they are confronting.

Each module contains a version for the therapist and a version for the caregivers and/or youth. The therapist version contains more information and detail about the topic. The youth and family versions are more streamlined and include a brief outline of the module. Prior to the session, the therapist should prepare by thoroughly reviewing the therapist version to ensure complete understanding of the topic and confidence in being able to effectively deliver the module and answer questions the youth and family may raise. Youth and/or family are prepared for the module session by being informed in a prior session (either individual or family) that they will be receiving a module. It is important to specify which module will be focused on and who will be receiving the module. The therapist also provides the youth and/or family members with copies of the module handouts so that they can review at home before the session and bring it back to use in the module session. Alternatively, clients can review the module handouts in the current session and ask the therapist to keep it for them for the following week. The therapist can also share the module with them electronically. The choice is given to the youth and/or family on which method they prefer.

During the module session, as the therapist leads the delivery of the content, the youth and/or family follow along with the handout. The therapist should check in often with the youth and/or family during the module to ensure that they are following along and are understanding the material. This is important because clients may feel embarrassed to stop the therapist or admit that they do not understand a concept. It is the responsibility of the therapist to make the family feel comfortable stopping the therapist for clarifications or questions throughout the module. Additionally, each module includes discussion questions for the caregivers and youth to break up the content and to ensure that they are understanding the material. These discussion points facilitate the process of connecting the module content to their everyday life. The therapist must balance the time spent on the discussion questions with continuing delivery of the module. When psychoeducational modules take more than one session, the therapist should make sure that this is not occurring because the module session is drifting and becoming an individual or family therapy session. Sessions dedicated to the delivery of psychoeducational modules should focus on delivery of the content and not be combined with a more traditional individual or family session. The reason is that a didactic process that focuses on sharing and discussing the specific topic of interest is more likely to lead to learning (i.e., with less processing of emotions) and more focus on understanding the role that the information or skills can play in the youth and/or family's daily lives.

Strategies to Increase Youth and Family Readiness When Delivering CIFFTA's Psychoeducational Component

- The therapist should emphasize that the youth/family are the experts of their situation.
- Emphasize that the therapist's role is to collaborate with the family in ways that they determine would be most helpful to them.
- Avoid judgment. If the youth and/or family sense that the therapist is judging them or lecturing them with information because they are deficient in a certain area, they may disengage and decide to discontinue services.

Generalizing the CIFFTA Module

Once a youth and/or family have received a module in its entirety, the therapist plans for the subsequent family or individual session, which will focus on generalizing the module to the client's everyday life. Module generalization is the process in which the therapist helps the caregiver(s) and youth to apply the knowledge/information learned in the module to the circumstances and situations that require change. To achieve this purpose, the therapist and family members highlight the three to four ideas from the modules that are most relevant to the youth and/or family and agree that these things will be a focus of future sessions. The therapist may need to work with the youth in an individual session before bringing the entire family together to focus on the topic. This preparation can help the youth be better able to identify their needs and feelings and then to express them in a healthy way to caregivers and other family members. Likewise, the therapist may meet with the caregivers alone, for example, after the Parenting module, to generalize the content to the family situations that are most problematic. For example, they may decide how to make a needed shift in how they communicate rules and monitor the youth. Once the caregivers are comfortable then all family members are invited to the family session to continue the implementation of the new parenting strategies.

In module generalization therapy sessions, the major themes that are initiated through the modules in a didactic manner (e.g., parenting practices, acculturation conflicts, emotion dysregulation, abandonment issues due to immigration-related separations) continue to be processed. In the didactic session, the focus may be on how the topic manifests itself in general and in many families. Once the generalization work begins, the family begins to talk specifically about their unique situation and how the topic plays out in their family. Using generalization, the youth and family implement the new adaptive behaviors on a regular basis and identify and modify any family patterns that impede or constrain the new desired behaviors. Interpersonal dynamics in the family (e.g., negativity, disengagement, triangulation, rejection, invalidation) that hinder good parenting practices or supportive parent–adolescent relationships are targeted for change. Subsequent family sessions should focus on shaping adaptive interactions using the new material. When a youth is engaging in substance use and they subsequently receive the Alcohol and Other Substance Use module, the individual sessions that follow may focus on returning to MI strategies to elicit from the adolescent their perspective on substance misuse and the information learned in the module. The therapist would collaborate with the youth to develop a goal in this area once the youth is motivated to make a change. The youth would also be prepared to share with family members in a family session what their goal is and how they would like the family to provide support. When conversations around substance use becomes more honest and truthful, trust can become reestablished in the family.

In the module generalization sessions, the therapist must be attentive to things like: Who supports or undermines whom? What is the level of negativity of the family and what triggers it? How do family members handle conflicts? What sequence of family member intrusion or disengagement keeps the problem going? One must also assess the rigidity or flexibility of these relationship patterns. In some cases, providing information and a new way of thinking about the family condition is sufficient to bring about new and more flexible interactions. In other cases, the family sessions focus on generalization and highlight the rigidity of family interactions. By making these problem interactions more visible, changes in the interactions become possible.

Addressing Challenges to Implementing CIFFTA's Psychoeducational Component

There are challenges and traps that can arise when delivering a module to a youth and/or family. These can also reduce fidelity to the model. Challenges are listed below along with tips on how to avoid these traps.

Drifting from a Module Session to a Therapy Session

It is common for youth and/or the family to want to share their own thoughts and questions related to what they are hearing in the module. This is valuable if the therapist maintains a focus on the material and does not allow complete deviation away from the content of the module. It helps anchor the material in their day to day experiences. If the session becomes a process-oriented therapy session, the focus on the material is lost, and the therapist cannot recover in time to present the rest of the relevant material. The therapist must redirect the youth and/or family to refocus on the module content. The therapist can say something like, "What you are sharing is important, and I want to come back to it in our next session. For now, let's continue to focus on this topic for today so we can see it in its entirety and decide how helpful it will be to you. In our next session we can focus fully on tying this into the important issues you are raising."

Therapist Is Not Prepared

If the therapist does not carefully review, understand, and become comfortable with the material presented in the module, they will have difficulty smoothly and seamlessly imparting the information to the youth and/or family. They may also inadvertently avoid checking in with the youth and/or family so that difficult questions are not asked. This means that the youth and/or family may not receive the full benefit of the module. Of course, sometimes there may be questions that the therapist cannot answer, and it is OK to say, "let me look into that and give you a more complete answer the next time we meet." But obviously the therapist will feel better if this is not a frequent occurrence. The comprehensive therapist version of the module content includes much more information than does the client handout, and that is designed to help the therapist feel prepared.

Youth and/or Family Are Not Prepared

If a youth or their family are not told ahead of time that they will be receiving a module in the following session, they may not engage in the session. This is especially true if the topic of the module is sensitive for the youth and/or family (i.e., substance misuse, immigration-related separation) or if their perception is that they are going to be told what to do in a dogmatic way. As previously stated, in the sessions prior to the module sessions, the youth and/or family should be prepared for what is planned for the following session. Remember that whenever possible, the selection of the module should be a collaborative effort, and this will improve the engagement of the family. If strong defensiveness or denial emerges, the therapist knows they should prepare the ground a bit more using MI.

Too Many Modules Are Selected

When families present with varied symptoms and issues, the therapist may feel that many modules would help the family. That may be true, however, overwhelming a family with modules is not helpful and may negatively impact their engagement. It is important for the therapist to balance each component of the CIFFTA treatment to maximize the impact for the family. It is best to prioritize three to four modules with the family and utilize the family and individual components of the model to process and focus with the family on addressing the most critical issues. If time permits during treatment, then the therapist can consider adding additional modules.

Therapist Is Not Checking In or Reviewing the Discussion Questions

To save time or to avoid delving into an area they are not comfortable with, the therapist may fail to check in with the youth and/or family or fail to ask the discussion questions throughout the module. It is important to check in and to ask the discussion questions as they are structured to help the family connect the content they are hearing to their daily lives. It is crucial that the adolescent and family have an opportunity to say that the content is highly relevant, not applicable, or not clear. It is not helpful if the client takes a very passive stance in the sessions and fails to do the work of connecting the dots. All along the way, the client must be active in anchoring the information to how they think and the situations around them. If family members do not see the practical value of what they are learning and when the information and skills will be useful, the content will be more easily forgotten or disregarded.

Expert versus Collaborator Therapist

If therapists conduct themselves in the manner of an expert who knows exactly what the youth or family needs to learn and do to fix their situation without family input, the family members may shut down and disengage. For youth and family to be open to receiving the module content, the therapist must reassure the youth/family that they are also experts of their situation, and that the therapist is there to collaborate with them on finding solutions and setting goals that will be most helpful to them. In the following box, you will see examples of the types of messages that empower families and those that can inadvertently disempower them.

How to Present the Psychoeducational Modules

How *not* to present the psychoeducational material	How to present the psychoeducational material
"I have noticed several problems in the parenting approach that you use and that we need to modify to make you better parents."	"Parenting an adolescent is particularly challenging in these complex times. I would love to go through some strategies with you and see if any of them seem to you like they can be helpful."

How *not* to present the psychoeducational material	How to present the psychoeducational material
"There is some information and knowledge that the family is lacking that I need to teach you all."	"Lots of families go through similar issues and there are some predictable patterns we often see and that you might find helpful hearing about. Would you be interested in covering these with me?"
"In this country we have more effective ways of approaching the problem with your son."	"Coming to a new country with different ways of handling things is complicated. I would love to talk about how this transition has been for you."
"The family's approach to your daughter's self-harm is not helping, there are better ways I can teach you."	"I would like to talk about what we know about kids who are self-harming in general and brainstorm with you about the best way to handle some of the challenges you have identified."
"Our team of experts on adolescents and families can tell you what you need to do to get this right."	"Our team has expertise in adolescents and families, but you have expertise on your adolescent and your family. By working together, we should be able to find some effective solutions."

Staying on Track

Use the CIFFTA Treatment Plan and the CIFFTA Postsession Therapist Self-Report of Adherence to stay on track with the psychoeducational work that you do with adolescents and families. Below are examples of questions that therapists can ask themselves while using CIFFTA's psychoeducational component. The questions can keep the work focused and on track.

- "Do I feel prepared to present the module fully and confidently?"
- "Did I work collaboratively with the adolescent and family in selecting the upcoming modules?"
- "Did I use the discussion points to anchor the content into their daily lives so that they can see the value to everyday situations?"
- "Did I deliver the module in a way that the family was active and not passively listening?"

- "Did I open the door to explore the role of culture in the content of the modules?"
- "Did I make sure that we did not drift into a therapy session that moved away from the main topic?"
- "Did I do the necessary work so as to identify how the module material will be generalized in future therapy sessions?"
- "Did I provide the opportunity for clients to say that they did not agree or that they did not feel comfortable with the strategies discussed?"

SUMMARY

In this chapter we have described the purpose of CIFFTA's psychoeducational component and the ways in which they facilitate the work of the individual and family therapy sessions. When used correctly, the psychoeducational material creates readiness to change and paves the way for the work that is done in future therapy sessions. By using a shared decision-making approach, the family can have a say in the topics selected and how they fit in with their conceptualization of the problem and their goals for treatment. We provided a brief description of the content of each module so that its purpose can be clearer and so that you can see how it fits in with the work we are often called upon to do. We also described the process that should be used in delivering the material, what it looks like when it is done well and, what it looks like when it is done poorly. Finally, we went into detail on the importance of using the subsequent individual and family therapy sessions to work on generalization of the material so that it becomes clear how the new information and skills should be used in daily life.

8

Case Examples Showing CIFFTA in Action

In previous chapters we described CIFFTA's individual, psychoeducational, and family components, and the tailoring approach designed so that the unique clinical and cultural characteristics of the youth and family are addressed in therapy. For diverse and marginalized clients who are known for underutilization of treatment, the therapy becomes more ecologically valid, relevant, and useful when it directly addresses their lived experiences. In this chapter we present four case studies that exemplify the use of CIFFTA and its components to address a variety of significant clinical, family, and culture-related issues. The key aspects of the case that exemplify the component and strategy used come from our own clinical experience, but we have modified less relevant facts (using composites from a variety of cases) to disguise true client identities. There is more complexity in each family than we can convey in brief case studies, but this should give the reader a good sense of how the CIFFTA components work together.

THE SUAREZ FAMILY

Carmen Suarez, a 15-year-old Latina, was referred to the CIFFTA program by her school counselor for symptoms of depression and poor school attendance. Carmen's mother called the program and stated that her daughter's school counselor was concerned because Carmen reported feeling sad and not wanting to go to school.

After completing an initial intake assessment, the therapist called the primary contact for the family, the mother. The therapist explained that all family members were invited to join the sessions. Carmen's mother reported that it might be difficult for Carmen's stepfather to attend due to his work schedule. The therapist felt that the mother did not have any concerns about stepfather attending sessions and would welcome his participation. The therapist asked the mother for permission to reach out directly to the stepfather to explain the program and to connect directly to him. This proved to be important because during the phone call with him, the therapist learned that the stepfather was reluctant to attend therapy. The therapist had the opportunity to answer his questions, address his concerns, and highlighted how important his perspective and views were to the therapy process. It is common for a stepparent to be unsure about the role they should play in childrearing. The therapist sent an important message about how his participation in the family would benefit his stepdaughter. Note that even if he had not attended due to having to work during those hours, his perspective on therapy and his role had already been modified. The stepfather decided he would like to attend at least once.

During the first session, the therapist met with the entire family first and then with the adolescent alone to complete the CIFFTA Clinical Interview (Chapter 4). It is a good strategy to meet with the adolescent alone during the first session to allow them the space to share anything that they might be reluctant to talk about with the entire family in early sessions. The therapist also takes the opportunity to elicit the adolescent's perspective on the issues the family is reporting on and to assure the youth that their perspective matters. Therapy was not necessarily Carmen's idea, so it is worth taking the time to engage her fully as a client.

The data from the intake assessment and the CIFFTA Clinical Interview were used to develop the CIFFTA Tailoring Report for the family. Their Tailoring Report highlighted elevated symptoms of youth depression, above-average family conflict, deficits in parenting practices and communication, and the presence of an immigration-related mother–child separation. Protective factors that emerged for the family during the CIFFTA Clinical Interview included family openness to treatment, motivation to improve family relationships, strong religious values, and church and community involvement.

The family system consisted of Carmen, the biological mother, stepfather, and a 7-year-old half-sister. During the CIFFTA Clinical Interview, the therapist learned that the mother immigrated to the United States alone while 6-year-old Carmen stayed in the country of origin with grandparents. Her biological father had contact with Carmen in the country of origin but stayed there when she left for the United States.

Carmen arrived in the United States 8 years after the separation and at the age of 14. It is interesting to note that in one of our research studies, the average separation for Latine families was 7 years and remarkably similar to Carmen's separation timeline (Mena et al., 2023). The family sought treatment 1 year after the reunification. The youth reported symptoms of depression including irritability, feeling sad, trouble sleeping, inability to concentrate, and lack of energy. The mother reported that Carmen had a difficult time getting out of bed in the morning and sometimes missed school several days per week. Ms. Suarez left to work early each day and could not take time in the morning to get Carmen out of bed and take her to school.

Unique Culture-Related Stressors Experienced by the Suarez Family

When Carmen was 6 years old, after her mother migrated to the United States, Carmen was cared for by her maternal grandparents. Once in the United States, the mother met her current husband and remarried. During the reunification, the adolescent expressed feelings of anger, hurt, and abandonment because she was left behind with little explanation. Only upon arriving in a new country did she find out that she had a stepfather and a half-sister. It was obvious that there had been limited communication about these important issues. The new family members who had a strong relationship and more extensive recent history with the mother not only made the reunion awkward, but it also made Carmen feel like an outsider.

Carmen also reported missing her grandparents, who had become her primary caregivers during the painful separation, as well as extended family members, friends, and her home. This is an often-overlooked *additional separation* from a loved one. The mother immediately stepped "back" into the maternal role and began to set rules for Carmen, but Carmen was not open to accepting these rules. Resuming a "normal" parent–child relationship was highly unlikely while Carmen was carrying the pain and anger resulting from being left behind when the mother came to the United States and being unprepared for the new family unit. There was a significant rupture in the relationship between Carmen and her mother and this negatively impacted their communication. When they did try to talk, things broke down quickly. Carmen felt that her mother did not care about her and that she had come to the United States to start a new life without her. Ms. Suarez felt that Carmen was being selfish and did not appreciate all that she had sacrificed by leaving her country alone with the hopes of providing a better life for her. This was certainly not the joyful reunion that Ms. Suarez was hoping for when she planned the reunification with her oldest daughter. In fact, the expectation that it should be a joyful time in their lives made the disengagement and the rupture in the relationship much more painful.

The Impact of Culture-Related Stressors on Symptoms

During the time that Carmen and her mother were separated, the adolescent progressed into adolescence and reached important developmental milestones. Upon reunification, Carmen was faced with a mother whom she resented and with whom she could not communicate. She also had to deal with a new country, a new language, new family members, and different customs and ways of living. The expectation that life should resume as if nothing had happened was not feasible. The loss of the person she considered "mother" while growing up, her grandmother, was also very painful and was not acknowledged. It was easy to underestimate how painful a second separation can be, especially given the closeness that can develop over an 8-year period during which Carmen was her most vulnerable. These stressors, and the lack of validation of the losses she had experienced, propelled her to experience symptoms of depression such as irritability, inability to sleep, feeling sad, and difficulty concentrating on her studies. Carmen felt isolated and had no interest in going to school, engaging with peers, or even communicating and interacting with her family.

Tailoring the CIFFTA Components to Meet the Needs of the Suarez Family

Early Phase of CIFFTA: Engaging, Joining, and Tailoring

The engagement efforts with the stepfather occurred prior to any formal sessions and was a significant first step toward creating the right environment for change. The first family sessions with the Suarez family focused on joining with Carmen, her mother and stepfather, and instilling hope that therapy could help them. While engaging with the family the therapist learned that whenever Carmen shared how hard it had been to be separated from her mother and how much she missed her grandmother, mother became defensive and frustrated. It is common to have parents ask that the youth look forward instead of "dwelling on the past." There were many misunderstandings between them and misconceptions about each other's feelings and behaviors. The therapist decided to have a session alone with the mother and stepfather focused on what the mother wanted her relationship with Carmen to look like. As the goal of having a healthy and open relationship with her daughter emerged, the therapist was able to highlight the discrepancy between that desire and the way the mother was shutting Carmen down when she became vulnerable and shared her feelings. Taking the time to solidify the mother's motivation for a strong relationship with her daughter and discussing how getting Carmen to share her feelings was the path to deepening the relationship, opened the door for more productive family sessions where she became more willing to listen to Carmen's pain and sense of lost time without becoming defensive. Having the stepfather's support for this approach meant he would not try to shut down Carmen when she expressed her pain and that he would help his wife to validate Carmen.

Early-phase individual sessions with Carmen focused on engaging and joining with the goal of forming a trusting relationship. MI was used to establish a collaborative relationship where Carmen felt heard and understood, and that her needs and goals for therapy would be prioritized and addressed. MI was also used to elicit the youth's own motivation to work on improving her symptoms, learning the customs and language in the United States, attending school, and on improving her relationship with her mother.

Tailoring Treatment Using the CIFFTA Psychoeducational Component

The CIFFTA Tailoring Report profile suggested that the psychoeducation modules most relevant for the Suarez family were the Immigration-Related Separation module (delivered to the family together), the Parenting module (delivered to the mother and stepfather alone), and the Depression module (delivered to the family together). The selection of the best-fitting modules for the Suarez family in collaboration with the family allowed the CIFFTA therapist to create a treatment plan that addressed the unique experiences and needs of the youth and family. The logic of the modules is that they provide the family with information and education so that the family is more ready to process the stressors and understand the impact they have on their family functioning and symptoms.

Because the separation between Carmen and her mother was at the core of many of the symptoms Carmen was experiencing and the ruptured mother–daughter relationship, the Separation module was the first module delivered to the family together. The mother, stepfather, and Carmen all attended the module session. It was important for stepfather to attend because he was an important part of Carmen's daily life and care. It was difficult for Carmen to accept him when she arrived, especially because Carmen felt that her mother had replaced her with a new family. His validation of her feelings could go a long way toward developing a strong relationship.

Starting with the Separations module was critical because an attempt to work on parenting, communication, and family relationships without addressing the separation, would be less likely to succeed and the family might become hopeless and disengaged from treatment. The Separations module normalizes the pain and sense of loss and resentment that often emerges during separations. It also normalizes the fact that it is difficult to face and discuss these painful experiences. Rather than framing the presenting issues as a result of pathology or dysfunction in the Suarez family specifically, the feelings and relational difficulties were presented as happening in many families who attempt the complex process of reunification after a long separation. In fact, we can honestly say to the family that if it had not been happening to many families, we would not have a stand-alone module on this topic. The content of the module helps to create a *readiness* for the family to process the separation, to share feelings related to the separation, and to clarify misunderstandings in later family sessions. The discussion questions included in the Separations module prompted Carmen and her mother to each share how they experienced the separation and to resist the natural and human tendency to become defensive.

The second module, the Parenting module, was delivered to the mother and the stepfather alone. For the Suarez family, the parenting module focused on providing the caregivers with education about the developmental stage the youth is in, the basics of effective communication, how to spend quality time together, setting limits, rules, and rewards, and learning how to validate the youth's feelings. These parents had to figure out how to be effective at parenting a 14-year-old from one day to the next. The transition from parenting a child to parenting an adolescent (and one with some anger at that) did not happen gradually as happens when a separation has not occurred. We often give the parenting module to the parent-figures alone so that they can talk freely about what has worked and what has not worked and so that they and the therapist can strategize about how to get the best possible response from the youth. It also allows for honest communication about how the parental team is working together and whether there are any disagreements about how to do the parenting. Any competing messages or undermining behavior can have powerful negative effects.

The Depression module was the third module that was delivered to the family together and provided them with education about the many aspects of depression and how symptoms manifest in the lives of individuals. The module also addresses stigma related to depression and normalizes the symptoms. This module can also be delivered to the youth and the caregivers separately to allow the youth space to share information privately. In this case, Carmen and her caregivers were open in their discussions about her struggles, so the therapist made the decision to provide the module to the family together.

Middle and Late Phases of CIFFTA: In-Depth Work on Individual and Family Functioning and Module Generalization

CIFFTA Family Component

Following the Separation module, family sessions became more honest, productive, and emotional (in a positive way). The therapist realized early on that Carmen and her mother needed to talk about the time they had been separated. Carmen had to tell her mother how painful the 8-year separation had been without her mother becoming angry and defensive. In some cases, an adolescent may feel the need to recount how difficult it was to spend Mother's Day at school and at home while not having a mother with them. In this case, her mother became able to validate Carmen's feelings about the separation and Carmen was able to hear and accept her mother's perspective about the loving and protective intentions that caused her to leave Carmen for those years. The mother's ability to listen and validate the youth's experience made a huge difference in the therapy and family process. In validation, you do not have to agree with every part of the other person's position, but you do need to allow them to have a position and honestly listen to it.

Healing the relationship between Carmen and her mother became a primary focus. Eventually, Carmen and her mother were able to hug for the first time in many years. At the same time, the stepfather was able to become closer to the mother–daughter dyad by experiencing this healing along with them. This is an important part of a successful therapy. Some therapists might limit the work to the mother and daughter and feel that the stepfather was not part of the immediate problem or solution. But from the perspective of having a new shared history, going through this healing together created a new set of connections in these three family members. Later, family sessions could include the half-sister and focus on establishing healthy communication and a caring relationship between the entire blended family. The special gift of having a sister can be highlighted in therapy. Working to strengthen the sibling subsystem can be highly effective and it is an often-overlooked part of family work.

Other areas that were the focus of family sessions were parenting and helping the family monitor and talk about Carmen's symptoms of depression. The mother and stepfather needed to learn how to effectively establish rules, monitor her behavior, and communicate with Carmen in an age-appropriate manner. This was new for Carmen as well. Family sessions that followed the delivery of the Depression module focus on generalizing the content from the module to their family. Learning how caregivers can help the adolescent during depressive episodes can be enormously powerful. This is an important step in the successful implementation of the CIFFTA components and reinforces how the three components work in a synergistic manner to achieve the goals of the family. Delivery of the general information without taking the next step of anchoring the new knowledge into everyday interactions is much less effective.

CIFFTA Individual Component

Individual sessions held after the Separations module provided Carmen with space to discuss her feelings about what she and her mother shared during the module and to prepare for the postmodule family session where the separation would be processed in more depth. The individual sessions were also utilized to generalize the information received via the Depression module with Carmen. The therapist monitored Carmen's symptoms of depression and identified daily triggers and her usual responses to these triggers. This provided the opportunity for the therapist and Carmen to work together on a plan to manage the situations and symptoms and to effectively seek family and other support as needed. Carmen's school attendance and performance were also areas focused on in the individual sessions.

Overall, the Suarez family received 15 sessions over approximately 14 weeks, receiving 7 family sessions, 5 individual sessions, and 3 psychoeducational module sessions. At the end of treatment Carmen's symptoms had improved, she was attending school and had a plan for improving her grades. The family's communication and connection improved significantly, and the therapist highlighted the gains they had made in therapy and the tools they now had at their disposal to continue to work on their relationships.

THE RODRIGUEZ FAMILY

The Rodriguez family is made up of a biological mother, maternal grandmother, and Juan, who was 16 years old. Juan was born in the United States. His mother immigrated to the United States with the maternal grandmother from a South American country 17 years before entering therapy. Juan had never met or had contact with his biological father, who remained in South America. The mother spoke little English and worked long hours through the afternoon and evening. Juan's grandmother lived with them and always helped Juan's mother with taking care of him. Juan spoke Spanish but preferred not to and became upset when his mother and grandmother pressured him to speak Spanish. Juan knew that he was of Latine decent, however, he considered himself to be American and felt little connection to his family's country of origin.

Juan was referred to the CIFFTA program by a care coordinator from a local community agency that helped connect families to resources they need, such as food, housing, medical, legal, and mental health services. Because the mother spoke little English and felt disconnected from local institutions, the role of the care coordinators and natural helpers was key to gaining the trust of the family, getting past the stigma associated with "treatment" and being willing to give the services a try. Juan's presenting problems included fighting at school, poor grades, anger management issues, and high conflict with his mother. During the initial sessions, the therapist met with the family and with the adolescent alone to complete the CIFFTA Clinical Interview.

The Rodriguez family's Tailoring Report highlighted elevated symptoms of conduct problems, poor school functioning, above average family conflict, deficits in parenting practices and communication, and a significant acculturation gap between mother and son. The acculturation gap measured using the Hispanic Stress Inventory and the acculturation scales reflected the fact that the mother identified highly with Hispanic cultural items and little with "Americanism" in terms of her language, customs, food preferences, and values. Conversely, Juan identified highly with "Americanism" items and little with "Hispanicism" items. This profile is quite different from one in which the individual has a *bicultural profile* and feels effective and comfortable in either culture or language. Protective factors that emerged for the family included motivation to improve family relationships and openness to attending therapy, youth engaged in extracurricular boxing activity, the mother having job security, having a supportive and engaged grandparent living at home, and the family feeling safe in their environment/neighborhood. We should note here that protective factors are often underappreciated by family members, and it is the therapist's job to highlight and enhance these important strengths.

Unique Culture-Related Stressors Experienced by the Rodriguez Family

Differences in acculturation between family members can negatively impact family relationships and can exacerbate adolescent problems. Although Juan's mother and grandmother immigrated to the United

States 17 years before, they had not incorporated American language, values, and beliefs. This does not always reflect a rejection of "Americanism" but reflects the fact that they may be intimidated by the language and system and feel they can make ends meet in a Latine enclave that does not offer opportunities to expand their experiences. Juan showed an "assimilated" acculturation response and felt disconnected from his family's culture of origin. He chose not to live in a bicultural fashion that used the best of the two cultures. We should note that many external factors can push the youth in this direction, including hearing constant anti-immigrant and anti-Latine messages. Juan's stance on this issue created conflict between him and his mother and grandmother. When Juan refused to speak in Spanish with them, they felt that he was rejecting them and their culture of origin and even looked down on them.

The grandmother had lived with Juan and his mother since he was born. She took on a parental role along with Juan's mother, who was a single parent, to support her daughter and grandson. Culturally, this is not uncommon and although helpful, it can present challenges as the grandmother vacillates between needing to act like a parent but having a desire to behave more as a grandparent. The mother and grandmother struggled with being on the same page in terms of parenting Juan and this caused conflict and arguments between them as well. As the family conflict intensified, Juan became less willing to speak in Spanish and make attempts at working through issues in the family. It is common for youth who are not as fluent in Spanish as they are in English to feel that speaking in Spanish makes them feel less powerful and more vulnerable. When there is conflict in the family, no one wants to feel powerless and vulnerable. The mother's lack of comfort with the host culture's language and routines reduced her involvement in Juan's school activities and with his peers. Juan's mother was completely disconnected from those areas of his life, and this created a greater divide between them.

The Impact of Culture-Related Stressors on Symptoms

The arguments in the family became more intense over the last four years as Juan entered adolescence. Juan felt stress at home and was resentful that his mother was barely around because she had to work so many hours and did not seem interested in his life. Although he was close to his grandmother as she had always been there for him and did her best to fill in for his mother, Juan became frustrated when she would tell him what to do and tried to impose limits. Although it was hard for him to admit, Juan was also angry that he had never met his father and felt abandoned. This caused friction between Juan's mother and Juan because a part of him blamed his mother for allowing that to happen. Juan's mother had never been able to openly discuss this with him, although it was a source of great pain for both of them. Some topics just felt taboo and best swept under the rug. Over time, Juan's anger became more intense and manifested itself in outbursts at home, school, and with peers. He had trouble with his schoolwork and lacked the discipline to complete assignments. Juan preferred to be out of the house to "get away from everyone and everything."

Tailoring the CIFFTA Components to Meet the Needs of the Rodriguez Family

Early Phase of CIFFTA: Engaging, Joining, and Tailoring

The mother, Juan, and the grandmother were invited to attend the family sessions. The therapist called each of them separately before the first session to connect with them and to let them know how important each of their perspectives was for the therapy. Sometimes grandmothers do not think they should be involved in treatment and there may be stigma around therapy, but the grandmother was key to a well-functioning Rodriguez family. This is especially true when grandmothers are part of the parenting subsystem and have caregiving duties that require good communication and agreement between the caregivers. During the initial phase of engagement, the therapist took extra time to instill hope. Juan and his mother appeared defeated and out of solutions. Instilling hope in families that feel they have failed and reached the end of the line is key to successful therapy. Too often an inexperienced therapist may label the family as disinterested and uncaring without appreciating how much they have been through and the efforts that have made over long periods to change the problem. The therapist took time to explain how family therapy could help them with their conflict and communication and normalized some of the stressors that had contributed to the conflicts. During these sessions, the therapist asked each of them to share their perspective, what was important for each of them, and took time to validate the mother, grandmother, and Juan. The therapist also highlighted the positive and loving messages that are the foundations of the relationships so that they rise above the conflict.

The therapist also took time to negotiate the language of the family sessions as it became obvious at the first session that Juan preferred to speak in English and the mother and grandmother continuously asked him to speak in Spanish so they could understand. Juan was reluctant to speak in Spanish as he was more awkward when speaking Spanish and felt uncomfortable. However, he agreed to speak in Spanish except for those instances when he wanted to say something that he felt he could better express in English. The mother and grandmother accepted this, and the therapist would help with the translation. As the relationship improved, Juan was more willing to take chances and accept the *vulnerability* that came with speaking Spanish and began to enjoy communicating more effectively. This change in interactions became important not only because it facilitated the therapy sessions, but also because it created a new interaction pattern that could be used at home to communicate directly and more effectively.

Engagement in the individual sessions with Juan focused on increasing his motivation to improve his grades; manage his emotions, particularly anger; and work on his relationship with his mother and grandmother. MI was used to facilitate this process. It was crucial to start at this point because it would have been difficult for the therapist to start the work in family sessions to resolve family conflicts and strengthen their relationships or to deliver the skills-based modules to Juan without him being motivated to make a change in these areas and having identified the reasons why *it was important to him* to make these changes.

Tailoring Treatment Using the CIFFTA Psychoeducational Component

Based on the information gathered from the intake and the CIFFTA Clinical Interview, the modules most relevant for the Rodriguez family were Parenting (delivered to the mother and grandmother), Emotion Regulation and Interpersonal Effectiveness Skills (delivered to Juan alone), and Acculturation (delivered to the family). The therapist began with the Parenting module and then followed with the Acculturation module. Then the skills-based modules, Emotion Regulation and Interpersonal Effectiveness Skills, were delivered to the youth.

The Parenting module was critical for Juan's mother and grandmother. Understanding Juan's developmental stage and his natural desire for autonomy as well as learning that effective parenting required consistency, rules, appropriate consequences, affection, quality time spent together, validating the youth's feelings, and good general communication were important for the mother and grandmother. It is also crucially important to ensure that the two caregivers are fully supporting each other and working through any differences that exist between them regarding parenting. An important part of the parenting discussion is allowing the mother and grandmother to share their values around family and parenting. Culture-related beliefs and values must be identified and honored even as their impact on parenting effectiveness is considered. These can include a need for strict hierarchy and respect, and valuing obligation to family over individualism. Validating the mother and grandmother's position was critical because the goal was not to have them abandon their values and beliefs but to help them find a balance between their needs and Juan's needs.

The Acculturation module was delivered to Juan, his mother, and grandmother together. This module provided them with information about acculturation and how it naturally occurs, different rates of acculturation often displayed by older and younger family members and how that difference between them could become stressful and impact family functioning and relationships. The module provided context for the different ways that the Rodriguez family members engaged in the acculturation process and allowed them to discuss the tension that existed because of these differences between them. Discussion questions within the module led them to discuss their differences in language preference and the mother's disconnection from Juan's school and peers and normalized these experiences. For example, many Latine parents are not oriented toward taking an active role in influencing teachers and other school personnel. What is sometimes labeled as *passivity* can really be a worldview that says that institutions should be respected by not intruding. The module provides education around this topic, and the discussion questions begin to help the family share their perspectives and values. This "sets the stage" for further work in family sessions where Juan and his mother could continue to share how their relationship has been impacted by the acculturation process, hear each other's perspective and experiences, and explore ways of moving toward a different level of understanding between them thus improving their communication and relationship. They could each consider making new decisions about how to expand their culture-related views and behaviors and consider the possible benefits of taking a more bicultural approach.

The skills-based psychoeducational modules that were delivered to Juan were Emotion Regulation and Interpersonal Effectiveness Skills. Juan was having difficulty managing his anger and had emotional outbursts regularly. This further harmed his relationship with his mother and impacted him at school when he became frustrated with his courses, teachers, and peers. It was important for him to start to notice when the anger was coming on, to name the emotion, to take a moment to think about what the best response could be to avoid hurting himself or someone else, and to strategize about alternative ways to cope and manage the moment. The interpersonal effectiveness skills helped Juan identify his needs and wants, learn strategies for communicating in an assertive not aggressive manner, to develop a plan that made it more likely he would get what he needed (e.g., including the timing of when to ask for things and how) and to avoid cutting off relationships and communications due to the way he expressed himself with others. The positive impact of both emotion regulation and interpersonal effectiveness were seen in family therapy sessions. This work led Juan to feel more comfortable identifying and communicating his need to know more about his father and reach out someday.

Middle and Late Phases of CIFFTA: In-Depth Work on Individual and Family Functioning and Module Generalization

CIFFTA Family Component

Early in therapy it became apparent that acculturation differences between Juan and his mother were driving much of the conflict, affecting the mother's ability to parent effectively, and affecting Juan's decision making and inability to control his emotions. His grandmother found it difficult to carry out consequences and set rules for her grandson. Furthermore, the mother was disconnected from every area of Juan's life, his friends, school, boxing activity, and did everything she could to avoid conflict with Juan. Juan was easily angered and in family sessions it was clear that they were unable to carry on a conversation for more than a few minutes before things would blow up. To decrease negativity, the therapist used reframes to allow the opportunity for them to consider a different way of interpreting what was happening between them. For example, Juan felt very hurt that his mother never asked about his boxing, helped him with school, or talked to him about his father. This made him vulnerable to explosions and outbursts. After the Acculturation module, the family sessions provided the context for Juan and his mother to process feelings related to difficulties acculturating to the United States. He was able to share this with his mother and she was able to listen and accept his feelings while he began to really listen to her experience as well. This validation touched Juan and over time he was able to soften his position and understand his mother's motivations and limitations.

Helping the mother and grandmother to be a more effective parental unit was also a central focus of the CIFFTA family work. There was room for improvement in terms of Juan's mother's ability to enforce rules, to communicate her expectations, and to become more involved in his school, boxing, and peer life. Family sessions allowed Juan and his mother to engage in respectful and productive discussions around her concern for his actions and her expectations. Over time, Juan was able to see how much his mother loved him, the negativity decreased, and their connection improved. This also allowed for the relationship between Juan and his grandmother to improve. As the mother took on more parenting responsibilities Juan responded well. Circularity tells us that sometimes it is not only how the caregivers implement their parenting strategies, but also how the adolescents interpret and give meaning to what the parents are doing. When youth feel that caregivers do what they do out of care and not out of some need to be controlling, the acceptance of the parenting behavior comes much easier. As the mother was more effective in the parenting role, the grandmother was able to support her daughter and enjoy her relationship with her grandson.

CIFFTA Individual Component

Individual sessions with Juan focused on setting goals for himself, generalizing the skills learned in the Emotion Regulation and Interpersonal Effectiveness Skills modules, and preparing Juan for more adaptive and effective interactions with his mother and grandmother in family sessions. After completing the skills modules, subsequent individual sessions with Juan focused on generalizing skills that were learned to specific situations in Juan's daily life. Using a diary card where he jotted down daily events, he was able to identify and name his triggers and emotions and make better decisions about what to do to soothe himself (boxing) without bringing harm to himself or his relationships. Through this process, Juan identified that he was angry at the fact that he did not have any contact with his father and that his father had never reached out to have a relationship with him. He and the therapist used the interpersonal effectiveness skills to practice how to talk to his mother in a way that would make her more likely to listen and consider his position. Juan had learned that she might not give him what he wanted but that effectively communicating with his mother would help him regain her trust and help them re-establish their relationship. These skills were also practiced in family sessions as Juan and his mother worked on improving their communications.

The Rodriguez family received treatment for approximately 14 weeks and attended a total of 22 sessions. Overall, they received 11 family sessions, 7 individual sessions, and 4 psychoeducational module sessions. At the end of treatment Juan, his mother and grandmother reported that although there were still some conflicts and misunderstandings at home, they were much better able to manage them without escalation. Juan began to show improvement in managing his emotions and outbursts and was committed to continuing to use the skills to avoid negative consequences for himself and his relationships with peers, school personnel, his mother, and his grandmother.

THE CRUZ FAMILY

The Cruz family was originally from Central America and had been in the United States for 10 years. Maria (14 years old), her biological mother and father, and younger brother (11 years old) lived in the home. Maria identified as a lesbian and although the parents were aware, they were having a difficult time accepting Maria's sexual orientation. Maria was referred to the CIFFTA program by a school mental health professional for engaging in self-harm behaviors (cutting and pinching) and symptoms of depression. Although her parents accepted the referral, when they initially called the CIFFTA program, the mother stated that they were not certain they needed the program because they felt that Maria was "exaggerating her symptoms." The family completed the intake assessment and in the next session the therapist completed the CIFFTA Clinical Interview. The CIFFTA Tailoring Report for the Cruz family highlighted above-average family conflict, youth engagement in risky behaviors, namely self-harm, elevated symptoms of depression, youth denial of the extent of self-harm behaviors, and parental rejection of Maria's lesbian sexual orientation. Protective factors that emerged included youth having a supportive peer group, youth connected to school community and doing well academically, youth having a healthy relationship with her younger brother, and parents being motivated to improve family functioning.

Unique Culture-Related Stressors Experienced by the Cruz Family

Maria's parents had a difficult time understanding mental health symptoms. They were raised into a very traditional worldview in Central America that believes that people with mental health issues are "crazy" and that it is not acceptable to share personal business with others. Their reluctance to "air dirty laundry in public" was one of the main reasons that they were reluctant to seek help for Maria. Part of it was also a tendency by some parents to minimize the significance of many types of self-harming behavior. This response is partly a defensive response given how helpless they feel. Maria had been raised hearing similar messages about mental health. She had a difficult time acknowledging her self-harm and described the cutting as "no big deal," "rarely happening," and "superficial." Furthermore, Maria identified as a lesbian and had disclosed this to her mother and father, but they felt that Maria was too young to know what she really wanted. They argued that she was being swayed by what she saw on social media, movies, and by her peers. They asked Maria not to share her orientation with their family and friends.

They were clearly worried about the reaction of extended family members who also tended to be traditional.

The Impact of Culture-Related Stressors on Symptoms

Because Maria's family had great difficulty understanding and accepting mental health issues, Maria did not feel that she could share her feelings with her parents. The stigma around emotional struggles and mental health treatment was powerful. The fact that the Cruz family would describe themselves as being *traditional* also impacted their discomfort with the topic of sexual orientation. The family was religious and were active in their church and friendly with the parishioners. The parents were concerned about how the church community would respond if they knew about Maria's sexual orientation. They were afraid of losing this otherwise supportive community. Maria did not feel accepted by her family and isolated herself at home and from extended family. These stressors propelled her to experience symptoms of depression such as isolation, hopelessness, lack of interest in previously enjoyable activities, difficulty sleeping, and self-harm behaviors. Maria had difficulty with emotional regulation and experienced moments where her anger and sadness where so powerful that she engaged in cutting and pinching behaviors to alleviate the intensity of her emotions.

Tailoring the CIFFTA Components to Meet the Needs of the Cruz Family

Early Phase of CIFFTA: Engaging, Joining, and Tailoring

The beginning phase of the family work focused on engaging and joining Maria, her mother, father, and brother. The therapist took time in this phase as the family was reluctant to participate. As a first step, the therapist spoke with both her mother and father and used some of the specialized engagement strategies designed for parents who may experience stigma around mental health treatment and who may have felt coerced into therapy by the school counselor. The therapist acknowledged a culture-related perspective that therapy was for "crazy people" and shared that this was a perspective shared by many people. By first showing an understanding for their worldview, the therapist was able to expand their perspective on who can benefit from therapy and engage the family to try a few sessions and then decide whether to continue. It helps to explain therapy in a way that fits best with the family's orientation. This may include describing therapy as coaching, advice, or fine-tuning parenting in a country with such different values and customs. It took time for the family to feel comfortable with sharing their personal lives and struggles with a stranger. It is important for the therapist to go slow, to validate their reluctance to participate in therapy, and to take the time needed to establish a collaborative spirit that allowed them to share their perspectives, cultural values and beliefs, and goals as a family. The therapist emphasized the point that the parents were the experts on their family and the therapist let them know that hearing from them was key to the process. When the therapist conveys that family values and perspectives will be an important part of therapy, parents are more likely to feel respected, understood, and open to participating in therapy. The therapist also normalized the issues that Maria and her family were struggling with and instilled hope that the CIFFTA program could address their family's needs. These were all necessary steps before moving on to specific family changes.

Maria entered treatment stating that she was participating because her school said she had to attend and not because she wanted therapy. Early phase individual sessions with Maria focused on engagement, joining, and increasing motivation to engage in treatment and to work on her self-harm behaviors. As the therapist used MI skills and established a collaborative relationship with Maria, an important goal emerged. Maria shared that she was having too many "aggressive moments" where she would become angry and lash out at her friends. It was hurting her friendships. This was particularly worrisome because we had identified a supportive peer group and school activities as protective factors for Maria. The aggressive reactions also emerged at home with her mother and father. Explosions at home sometimes led her to cut because she could not control her anger or because she was ashamed of her actions. The ability to identify and safely discuss these patterns opened the door for the therapist to introduce the psychoeducational skills modules, that is, Emotion Regulation and Distress Tolerance, as ways to help her manage the moments when her emotions felt out of control.

Tailoring Treatment Using the CIFFTA Psychoeducational Component

Based on the information from the CIFFTA Clinical Interview and the Tailoring Report, the modules most relevant for the Cruz family were the Self-Harm module (delivered to the family together), the Gender Identity and Sexual Orientation module (delivered to the family together), the Distress Tolerance module (delivered to Maria alone), and the Emotion Regulation module (delivered to Maria alone). The Parenting module (delivered to the parents alone) is generally always delivered to caregivers and was the module that the therapist delivered first.

The Parenting module focused on providing the parents with

education about the developmental stage Maria was in, information on how to communicate effectively and spend quality time together, information on setting limits and rules, and rewards, and learning how to validate the youth's feelings. The therapist encouraged the mother and father to share their values and beliefs around family and parenting and validated their views. This was a necessary first step that would facilitate the delivery and later generalization of the Self-Harm and Gender Identity and Sexual Orientation modules.

The first skills-oriented psychoeducation module that the therapist completed with Maria was the Distress Tolerance module. Maria was actively cutting, and the module focuses on developing a tailored plan to use in the moments when emotions become so overwhelming that they were not manageable. The idea of this module is to teach skills that help the youth to realize that the emotion will not last forever, and to survive the moment without hurting themselves or others. Maria was highly engaged in the module work and was willing to try several strategies to find the ones that would most likely work for her and keep her from self-harming. The step of ensuring the right fit for Maria was important because different practices work best for different individuals. Maria was able to identify strategies related to the sense of touch worked best for her. She even ordered stress balls on Amazon because she found that squeezing the foamy ball helped her cope when an emotional surge occurred. Maria also used ice cubes on her forehead and arms as the cold feeling on her body helped as well. The Emotion Regulation module was used next, to help Maria learn skills to help her identify, name, and accept her emotion when a surge occurred and to take time to choose a response that would be effective. Helping Maria learn skills to regulate her emotions allowed her to manage her reactions, utilize her distress tolerance coping, and reduced the need to self-harm.

The Self-Harm module and the Gender Identity and Sexual Orientation module were delivered to the family via video format in session with the therapist present. Because all family members were aware of both the self-harming behaviors and of Maria's sexual orientation, the therapist made the decision to deliver the modules to the family together. These video modules were developed as part of a new computer hybrid CIFFTA that is presented in Chapter 10. The video modules include questions for family members to give their perspective on the content they are viewing. The Self-Harm module covers content such as the definition and rates of self-harm, interpersonal and intrapersonal triggers to the behaviors and ways to respond to the triggers, and how therapy can help reduce self-harm behaviors. The Cruz family responded well to the module and Maria's parents were able to learn that self-harm is much more common than they thought and to understand the kinds of stressors that are linked to self-harm. When family members learn to manage their anxiety and understand that the behavior is a result of distress and not merely manipulative or attention-seeking behavior, they are better able to respond effectively. It was helpful for Maria to hear the information and it helped her feel validated and not "crazy."

The Gender Identity and Sexual Orientation video module was developed in collaboration with a local association that has expertise and provides LGBTQ+ relevant courses and education to families, individuals, and organizations. The module is composed of three recordings that explore the topic of sexual orientation with youth and families. The first video is about the coming out process, the second video is about stigma and stressors often experienced by LGBTQ+ individuals, and the third video is about support and empowerment for youth and families. The videos are powerful because the narrators are youth and their family members who have gone through the coming out process and they very honestly share their personal experiences, struggles, and successes they encountered on their journey. Maria and her parents watched the videos together with the therapist. They all responded with heavy emotion. Family sessions following the module focused on processing their emotions.

Middle and Late Phases of CIFFTA: In-Depth Work on Individual and Family Functioning and Module Generalization

CIFFTA Family Component

Mid- and late-phase family sessions with the Cruz family focused on identifying important family interactions and patterns that needed to be addressed. The interactions between Maria and her parents were negative and laden with conflict. It was difficult for the mother and father to acknowledge that she had symptoms of depression that contributed to self-harm behaviors and required treatment. When family members feel that the distress is exaggerated, or that behaviors are designed only to get attention, or to manipulate other people, they do not respond in a supportive or effective way. All these reactions keep the parents from getting to understand the youth's distress and to help them during difficult times. The parents' discomfort with their daughter being a lesbian led them to communicate with Maria in a way that made her feel rejected and alone. It should be noted here that some individually oriented therapist may disagree with some very traditional family values (which they may feel are rejecting and damaging the youth) and decide that it is better to leave the family out of therapy (to avoid additional hurtful comments) and to work with the adolescent alone. We strongly disagree with this position. The fact is that the adolescent will still return to the home and the family, and the harmful and painful messages will be unchanged. We believe strongly that it is much better to take responsibility for reshaping the family perspective and messages rather than to accept them as unchangeable. Of course, this requires that the therapist not reject the family and their views outright but instead validate the parents' right to their worldview as they simultaneously try to expand the perspective. This family work can occur at the same time as the therapist works individually with the adolescent to enhance resilience. CIFFTA works on change from both sides of the circular relationships.

Family sessions after the Self-Harm module helped the family process beliefs and values that kept the parents from accepting their daughter, identify the origins of her mother and father's beliefs, withhold judgment, validate one another, and express love and support for one another. After the Gender Identity and Sexual Orientation module, family sessions focused on Maria's sexual orientation and her mother and father's discomfort with the topic as well as the complications that came with their religious views. Maria shared with her parents what it feels like to not be accepted by them, and her mother and father were encouraged to share their perspective and values in a respectful and noninjurious manner. The family was able to hear each other and acknowledge each of their values around this issue. Although it was difficult for the parents, they heard Maria and let her know that although they were not ready to accept her identifying as a lesbian and that they worried about how the family would respond to her, they loved her, would never reject her, and were open to continuing the conversations. It helps when the therapist asks the adolescent whether it took them time to understand and accept who they were. This normalizes the fact that the family may also need time to process it successfully. Part of the work with families is helping them understand how change and healing takes time.

CIFFTA Individual Component

Mid- and late-phase individual sessions with Maria focused on monitoring her self-harm behaviors, generalizing the Distress Tolerance, Emotion Regulation, Gender Identity and Sexual Orientation, and Self-Harm modules, and preparing for interactions with her parents in family sessions. For example, when generalizing the distress tolerance skills that were learned in the module, the therapist worked together with Maria to identify other areas of Maria's life and situations where the same skills could be used. These included difficult interactions with her parents and peers. The therapist monitored her self-harm behavior by asking if any cutting had occurred in the previous week and reinforcing the use of the distress tolerance plan that had been established while completing the module. The use of diary cards can be quite effective in terms of documenting urges and triggers and identifying barriers to the use of skills. Halfway through treatment, Maria had stopped cutting. After the family completed the Self-Harm module and the Gender Identity and Sexual Orientation module, the therapist used individual sessions to provide Maria with a space to share her emotions, her feelings of rejection, and her not being understood by her family. The therapist worked with Maria to shape the communications she wanted to have with her parents during family sessions. The preparation with Maria during individual sessions facilitated the work in family sessions.

The Cruz family received treatment for approximately 18 weeks and a total of 32 sessions. Overall, they received 13 family sessions, 11 individual sessions, and 8 psychoeducational module sessions. At termination, Maria reported that she had not engaged in self-harm since week 5 of treatment. The family had made progress on communication and the mother and father had gained a better understanding of Maria's self-harming behavior. They were better able to validate her feelings. While the mother and father made headway in accepting Maria's sexual orientation, they acknowledged that it was still difficult for them. This is normal and the therapist validated their feelings and acknowledged the progress they had all made.

THE SANCHEZ FAMILY

Ramon Sanchez, 17 years old, was referred to the CIFFTA program by a juvenile services case manager for substance use, mainly marijuana and alcohol. Ramon had been caught skipping school and smoking marijuana behind a nearby grocery store by the school police. Ramon was referred to the Juvenile Services Division. Because it was the first time that Ramon had any legal trouble, the court referred him to a diversion program that required him to attend counseling, attend school, and complete community service hours. If Ramon complied, his record of the incident would be cleared in the system. Ramon lived with his biological mother and two brothers (20 and 22 years old). Ramon was born in the United States while his parents were from Cuba and had immigrated to the United States over 20 years ago. Ramon's parents were divorced. Although his father was present in his life, Ramon never had a close relationship with him, and their relationship was very conflicted. Although Ramon was close to his brothers, they also argued frequently because they did not agree with Ramon's choices or the path he was on. It was important that the brothers were nudging Ramon away from self-destructive behavior and not toward it as often happens when older siblings are part of the risk factor profile (e.g., providing access to drugs or criminal behavior).

The first sessions focused on completing the CIFFTA Clinical Interview. These data, along with those from the intake assessment were used to create the Sanchez family's CIFFTA Tailoring Report. The Tailoring Report showed elevated symptoms of conduct problems, depression, poor school functioning, engagement in risky behaviors, namely alcohol and marijuana use, and high family conflict. Protective factors that emerged for the family included strong relationships with siblings that were living a healthy life, both mother and the siblings were motivated to help Ramon, youth had some insight into his behaviors and actions, youth showed respect for family and others, and the family was financially stable and living in a safe environment with strong neighborhood connections.

Unique Culture-Related Stressors Experienced by the Sanchez Family

Ramon felt that he was targeted by the school police because of his Latine background. Ramon felt that the school police treated him, and his friends differently than they treated the "White kids" at school who were also using drugs. His peer group was also involved with drug use and in the past, they had been cited for trespassing and skipping school as well. Throughout his schooling, Ramon reported being bullied for being a Latine with brown skin and speaking with an accent despite having been born in the United States. During the intake assessment, Ramon expressed that if he were White, he would not have been turned over to Juvenile Services. Although Ramon's mother understood what he felt and thought that this might be true to some degree, she told Ramon that he had to stay out of the spotlight, follow the rules, and avoid trouble.

The Impact of Culture-Related Stressors on Symptoms

Ramon reported that he did not feel comfortable anywhere in his life, not home, school, or socially. His experience with being bullied and discriminated against for looking and speaking the way he does has been a constant stressor. The intensity of these stressors drove Ramon to seek out peers who were angry, rebellious, and not good influences. He began to use marijuana and drink alcohol at age 15 and he stopped caring about school and his grades. Ramon reported feeling down and depressed, having difficulty concentrating and sleeping, feeling anxious and worried, and being unable to relax. Things at home were conflictual and Ramon and his mother fought often. His relationship with his brothers had also become strained and he was not on speaking terms with his father. Ramon reported feeling angry all the time and wanting to run away.

Tailoring the CIFFTA Components to Meet the Needs of the Sanchez Family

Early Phase of CIFFTA: Engaging, Joining, and Tailoring

Initially the therapist made separate phone calls to each brother, father, and to the mother for engagement purposes. The therapist shared that therapy would be much more successful if they were involved and shared their perspectives. Everyone agreed to attend the sessions except for Ramon's father. He stated that he would try to attend a session at some point but that he was not willing to participate initially. Although the therapist was unsuccessful at bringing the father in, the message about his important role in the family and being welcomed into treatment was conveyed. The early-phase family sessions focused on engaging and joining Ramon, his mother, and his brothers. The initial sessions focused on instilling hope that therapy could help Ramon and the family with their relationship difficulties and with the presenting problems. The therapist elicited each family member's perspective, validated their feelings and experiences, and asked them to identify their goals for therapy. Confidentiality was discussed together with all family members present so that everyone was clear and comfortable with the limits of confidentiality.

Early individual sessions focused on engaging and joining with Ramon. This phase was extremely important because to authentically join with Ramon, the therapist needed to differentiate themselves from the Juvenile Services Division and Ramon needed to feel that the CIFFTA program was not merely an extension of the "punishing" system that was "forcing" him to attend. The therapist punctuated that the program staff was there to help Ramon with whatever he decided was important to focus on. Even if the system required treatment, Ramon was told that he could select a different program and therapist. This allowed Ramon to *choose* to work with *this* therapist. The therapist expressed hope that he would choose to stay with this program and give them an opportunity to help. The decision was his and the therapist was there to collaborate with him to help him meet the goals that he defined for himself. The therapist also evoked Ramon's perspective on his situation and validated Ramon's sense that Brown and Black youth may get into this system more easily and acknowledged that having a good lawyer helps many youth avoid the system.

The therapist used MI to increase Ramon's readiness to improve his relationship with his mother and brothers, manage his emotions, and consider the value of discontinuing or reducing his substance use. Although Ramon recognized that things were not going well in several areas of his life, he seemed uncertain about what he could do differently or how he could go about making changes. MI strategies such as pros and cons, reflections, open-ended questions, looking forward and backward, and readiness scaling were implemented to help resolve his ambivalence. After several sessions, Ramon was able to communicate that he wanted to make changes because he did not want to lose his relationships with his brothers, and he did not want to continue to engage in the types of behaviors that put him at risk for getting arrested. It became evident to the therapist that Ramon was motivated to learn how to manage his anger, anxiety, and stress. Ramon was able to see how the difficulty controlling his emotions was connected to his substance misuse and how it was affecting him physically and hurting his grades. He also recognized the emotional toll it was taking on his mother. Even his brothers were concerned and were trying to help him turn his life around before things deteriorated further. At this point, Ramon's motivation to make changes had increased significantly so it made sense to transition to the next phases of the CIFFTA treatment.

Tailoring Treatment Using the CIFFTA Psychoeducational Component

Based on the CIFFTA assessments and Tailoring Report, the modules that were most relevant for the Sanchez family were the Parenting module, including the Single Parenting component, the Alcohol and Other Substance Use module, the Discrimination module, and the Emotion Regulation and Interpersonal Effectiveness Skills modules. The Parenting module was the first module delivered to the mother alone. Although the father was invited to the session, he did not attend. Ramon's mother had become paralyzed for fear of Ramon's reactions and was not effectively providing structure, monitoring, and leadership. It is common with an explosive adolescent that the parent steps back from important parenting practices. The Parenting module helped the mother gain confidence and the tools she needed to re-establish herself as an effective parent. Of course, it is critically important that at the same time the therapist was helping the youth better understand the mother's parenting and loving intentions. The Alcohol and Other Substance Use module was important because Ramon's misuse of marijuana and alcohol was an important part of the presenting problem. They each (the mother with the brothers together and

Ramon alone) received the module in a didactic manner to allow for more open discussions, especially for Ramon. The module provided information/education about marijuana and alcohol and their impact on the body, brain, and emotional symptoms. Given that marijuana use is more prevalent and accepted, the conversation often focuses on its impact on the developing adolescent brain and how the impact for youth and adults may be different. Once everyone in the family received the module, the subsequent family sessions focused on helping the mother, Ramon's brothers, and Ramon discuss his drug and alcohol use, the effects on his physical and mental health, and how it was hurting his motivation for school and relationships with his family. The family also received the Discrimination module together. The module defines discrimination, including how it can impact mental and physical health and relationships. Discussion questions within the module help family members begin to think about experiences they have had with discrimination and how it has affected them and their family members. This module was important for Ramon and his family given his previous and current experiences of being treated poorly because of the way he looks and speaks and the stress this caused him. Families do not always take the time to discuss these issues, ways they can support each other, and share perspectives on how to thrive in that context. The successful processing of these issues helps to avoid the internalization of these harmful views.

The first skills modules that were delivered to Ramon were the Emotion Regulation and Interpersonal Effectiveness Skills modules. Ramon was having difficulty managing his anger and had emotional outbursts regularly. This further harmed his relationship with his mother and brothers and impacted him at school when he became frustrated with his courses. The interpersonal effectiveness skills helped Ramon learn strategies for communicating in an assertive rather than an aggressive manner and to avoid bringing conflict to his relationships because of the way he expressed himself. After completing the modules in the subsequent individual sessions with Ramon, the therapist focused on generalizing skills that were learned to specific situations in Ramon's daily life where the skills could be used.

Middle and Late Phases of CIFFTA: In-Depth Work on Individual and Family Functioning and Module Generalization

CIFFTA Family Component

Once the key family members were engaged, the family sessions focused on improving communication between them, managing conflicts, and generalizing skills learned in the psychoeducational modules. The first generalization work focused on what was learned in the Parenting module. Helping Ramon's mother to be a more effective parent was a central focus of the CIFFTA family work. Initially, sessions were held with the mother alone and focused on generalizing the parenting skills the mother had gained to her relationship with Ramon. His mother was afraid to enforce rules and to communicate her expectations to Ramon for fear that he would lash out and there was a risk he would run away. She was scared because he had fallen in with the wrong crowd and was using drugs and drinking. The mother did not trust Ramon, which also exacerbated their conflicts. In subsequent sessions with Ms. Sanchez, Ramon, and his brothers present, the mother shared her expectations with Ramon, rules, and consequences. It is important in these sessions that the therapist reduce the temperature of the arguments, refocus on the positive intentions behind the mother's words and requests, and that each person be validated. Family sessions allowed Ramon and his mother to engage in discussions around their conflicts and how things would break down between them. These conversations continued to be the topic of family sessions for some time as change was slow and Ms. Sanchez needed the support to remain consistent. Over time, Ramon was able to see how much his mother loved him and why she had lost trust in him. Although his father never attended a session, Ramon was able to talk with his mother about his anger toward his father and the therapist intervened by using reframes and assisting Ms. Sanchez in validating and supporting Ramon. The use of the siblings was also important. Siblings are often underutilized resources in family therapy. They can be a great resource because they have shared much of the history, including family experiences, immigration experiences, and discrimination. Caring and successful siblings can offer strategies for surviving in a tough world, offer support, and offer strategies for dealing effectively with the parents during their most difficult moments. Successful older siblings are often experienced as "disapproving and siding with the parents" so any work that can bring them alongside the identified client to provide support and mentoring can be immensely powerful. Strengthening the sibling subsystem can go a long way in the life of the adolescent.

Over time the negativity in the family decreased, and their relationship improved dramatically. The opportunity to have the family interact with one another was effective in helping the therapist identify areas in which their interactions and communication could be strengthened. The work then shifted to improving their communication patterns and helping shape their responses to conflict and emotions. The caring and protective intentions behind the communications were constantly highlighted.

The family sessions were also used to generalize the Discrimination module and Alcohol and Other Substance Use module together. It was important to help Ramon's mother and brothers learn how to talk to the adolescent about discrimination and risky behaviors such as substance use. The family sessions that followed the modules allowed them to effectively share their feelings on these subjects and to talk about how they impact the family. The therapist shaped the communications by coaching them to increase positive statements, enhance connections, and to validate each other's feelings and perspectives. This openness allowed the mother the opportunity to express her love, caring, and support of Ramon and to understand his vulnerabilities and stressors. Ramon's brothers also expressed their support. Over time, Ramon was able to reciprocate and express his love and affection for his mother and brothers. Ramon better appreciated the reasons for his mother's concern, fears, and the necessary changes in parenting. The therapist conducted several family sessions with just Ramon and his brothers (sibling subsystem sessions) to solidify their connection and build on the strength of their relationship.

CIFFTA Individual Component

Middle- and late-treatment individual sessions focused on monitoring risky behaviors, generalizing the substance use module and skills modules to his daily life, and preparing Ramon for family interactions in family sessions. The therapist focused discussions on Ramon's peer group and risky behaviors. When he entered treatment, Ramon was drinking on the weekends at parties and was smoking pot after school about three times per week and on the weekends. Because Ramon was sufficiently motivated to change his behavior, the therapist focused on collaborating with Ramon to develop a plan to reduce his use with the goal of discontinuing it all together. The therapist periodically checked in with Ramon on how the plan was going, what his triggers were, and how he could work through barriers that got in the way of his staying clean. The therapist and Ramon also discussed how Ramon could establish peer relationships that were healthier and supportive of success. Discussions related to relapse prevention were included as treatment progressed and Ramon achieved milestones of staying clean for a period of a month. In the individual sessions, Ramon was encouraged to share (and practice sharing if necessary) his progress, triggers, and barriers with the family during family sessions. The therapist helped Ramon practice what he would say and how he would say it as well as preparing effective responses for different reactions that family members might have. Helping Ramon to react effectively in the context of family members who are reacting badly is an outstanding opportunity for the practice of skills.

The generalization of the Discrimination module, the Emotion Regulation and Interpersonal Effectiveness Skills modules were important topics to discuss in the individual sessions. Ramon was able to identify his anger and make better decisions about what to do to soothe himself without bringing harm to himself or his relationships. The therapist and Ramon also used the interpersonal effectiveness skills to practice how to talk to his mother in a way that would make it more likely she would listen and consider his position. Ramon had learned that she might not give him what he wants but that effectively communicating with her would eventually help him regain her trust and help them re-establish their relationship.

The Sanchez family received treatment for approximately 16 weeks and attended a total of 28 sessions. Overall, they received 12 family sessions, 9 individual sessions, and 7 psychoeducational module sessions. At termination, they reported better communication and a stronger relationship with each other. Ramon had a better sense of his triggers and how to manage his anger and substance use. Although he occasionally had a slip, he remained committed to achieving abstinence and following his relapse prevention plan.

SUMMARY

In this chapter we described four adolescents and families presenting to therapy with quite different profiles and clinical needs. We hope that these cases help to illustrate not only the type of stressors that youth and families experience but also how these conditions create ruptures in family relationships and fuel symptoms. We attempted to show that there can simultaneously be risk and protective factors at the level of the individual, the family, and the larger context. We have also demonstrated how CIFFTA strategies and tools can be used to gradually tailor the treatment to the unique family needs, increase motivation to change, increase support and protection, decrease negativity and conflict, and shape interactions so that they are more adaptive and supportive of the well-being of all family members.

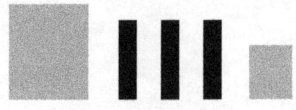

BROADER CLINICAL CONSIDERATIONS

III

BROADER CLINICAL CONSIDERATIONS

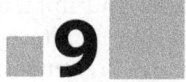

Training, Implementation, and Sustainability

with Alejandra C. Santisteban

Developers of evidence-based treatments (EBTs) were hit by a proverbial ton of bricks by reports outlining the difficulties in transporting available EBTs into practice (Institute of Medicine, 1998, 2007). Although some teams have been very successful at training, coaching, and dissemination of their EBTs, we have also learned that the roads to the front lines of practice are treacherous and often lead EBTs over a cliff, never to reach their intended destination or sustainment. Sometimes it appeared as though a traveler needing help to arrive at a difficult-to-reach destination, expected to be guided by Google Maps only to find out that all they had was a wrinkled and outdated paper map. One expert on effective implementation and sustainability described many of our outdated dissemination plans as *spray and pray* (Blasé, 2007). Furthermore, the teams that have succeeded in their sustainment efforts require considerable levels of engagement and resources over long periods of time.

We do not have the equivalent of an easy-to-use Google map for adoption and implementation of EBTs and our practices are far from being user friendly or affordable. Backer (2000) suggested that to reduce the research to practice gap, it might be wise to conduct a "gap analysis" that involves a rethinking of the processes and practices we depend on

---

Alejandra C. Santisteban, MPH, Denver, Colorado.

to disseminate and transport EBTs. The field can benefit from evidence-based and cost-effective methods for training and implementation that support therapist mastery of new skills and that facilitate sustainability. Just as innovations have led to more effective treatments, innovations must lead to evidence-based training, coaching, support, and implementation processes and tools.

This chapter describes the training and implementation challenges and the promising approaches for closing the gap. We begin by presenting innovations related to training and mastery of a new EBT (e.g., learning and mastering systemic competencies and engagement of family members). We discuss the ways in which an online training platform can be superior to traditional training events for *individual practitioners* (e.g., using simulation to increase the practice of new skills and providing expert feedback). Then, we present innovations pertaining to implementation and sustainment of EBTs *at the agency level* (e.g., increasing agency readiness, reducing staff turnover and cost). We will show how our online learning platform with simulation and expert feedback can help you gain mastery and confidence and, at a larger agency level, how it can be used to better train, coach, and support an entire workforce.

RETHINKING TRAINING AND MASTERY OF THERAPY COMPETENCIES

Training is key to improving provider knowledge and skill in the delivery of an EBT, but there is disagreement on what constitutes the most effective training methods (Powell et al., 2013). As a practitioner, you may have been exposed to many novel treatments, but you know that integrating that treatment into your regular practice is a complex endeavor. This is especially true when the treatment you are accustomed to delivering is qualitatively different from the new treatment. New concepts and techniques may seem interesting, innovative, and intuitive, but when you try to integrate them into complex clinical situations, the road can be a bumpy one. It is normal for lots of implementation questions to emerge following exposure to a new treatment.

Traditionally, training in a new EBT consists of a multiday live training event with a model expert who introduces the trainee to core concepts and attempts to sprinkle in role plays whenever possible. Past training in CIFFTA has been no exception. When the training is well-planned, learners typically report high satisfaction, but there are predictable drawbacks to this traditional approach. The first drawback is that it can promote passive learning because except for occasional role-play activities, learners often listen to a series of presentations. Using the lecture format there is little opportunity to process the information, to assess what is being learned, to adjust to the individual needs of the learner, and to practice the new skills. A second drawback is that this type of training can be expensive because of the expert time needed. Furthermore, because the expert's time is utilized in the teaching of basic concepts, the bulk of the training dollars are often allocated to this initial training process and resources are unavailable for the ongoing coaching and support needed to implement and sustain the new treatment. A concept that is challenging the front-loading of the expert time comes from the *reverse-classroom* framework (Bergmann et al., 2012; Bennet et al., 2012), in which the expert or lecturer time is best used for more advanced work and not for teaching the basics. Finally, this traditional approach is somewhat limited and rigid in that if a trainee gets sick or has a clinical emergency, they may miss key portions of the training completely. As we will see later in the chapter, this is also the case when an agency experiences staff turnover soon after the training event occurs, and new staff require training.

THE PROMISE AND CHALLENGES OF ONLINE TRAINING

For the reasons outlined above, online therapist training methods are gaining attention, and they have been shown to increase knowledge, skill, self-efficacy, and rates of training completion (Roh & Park, 2010). Online platforms can be an effective way to train clinicians on the basic concepts (Jackson et al., 2018). Online learning platforms can deconstruct learning material into meaningful "chunks" or "bite-size" learning opportunities that can stand alone, be followed by quizzes, and enriched with multimedia demonstrations. Unlike in person learning situations that involve large groups, an online platform allows the learner to decide on the additional demonstrations and practice they need. In effect, they can drive the training.

There are additional promising possibilities that come with online learning. One is that it can benefit from cost-effective and realistic simulations. Authentic clinical simulations are useful, engaging, and effective means of facilitating trainee learning of mental health interventions (Murray, 2014). The use of simulations allows you to interact with patients in a safe, realistic online environment. You can learn how to join, assess, and intervene with individual, couples, and family units representing a variety of clinical situations. This can help you develop and practice new ways of addressing client problems without the stress and pressure of having this first experience be in front of a real family. One of the clearest indicators of the usefulness of clinical simulations is that our trainees often report becoming anxious seeing conflict emerge in the family simulations, especially when they are expected to deliver an intervention. Experiencing this stress and anxiety when confronted with a simulated complex clinical situation and figuring out how to handle the situation more effectively, is great practice prior to being in front of a real family. We have found that the customizable characters in a simulated session enhance clarity using a show, don't tell approach, with scenario-based instruction and demonstrations.

A second benefit of using an online platform has to do with just-in-time learning. Many learners enjoy having information readily available and having the option to pull up "how to" articles as they are figuring out software or an answer to a random question. As a result, they are used to learning as they go, looking up information as they need it. The learning and development response to this current way of finding information is the just-in-time (JIT) learning and support format. JIT is facilitated by information that is available on demand, around the clock, and easily accessible through mobile devices (laptops, tablets, phones). As a learner, it would be highly attractive to be able to access material, including short "how-to" videos demonstrating important family intervention techniques that a therapist might use. Having access to such a demonstration is also highly valuable as a refresher during the implementation process.

There are, however, challenges that have emerged with online training (Harrison, 2021) that must be addressed if this approach is to be successful. One challenge is having more limited connections to other learners and trainers, resulting in a reduced sense of community. Learners like to have contact with peers and the opportunity to discuss clinical work. This may be missing in online training and important to some learners. As we will discuss later in the chapter, the integration of peer learning networks is one approach that can offset this drawback. Second, when online platforms are not designed to be engaging and interactive, there is the potential for high rates of dropouts and poorer retention. It is no easy task to make online platforms interactive and stimulating. Third, in our work with community-based treatment agencies, we have heard of online systems that introduce new treatment options in a cursory way and that do not lead therapists to be confident during the implementation phase. These agencies often report that the therapists use the systems but they do not significantly impact practice. There is great variability among online platforms, and it is a mistake to think that the considerable limitations of the first generation of online platforms are inevitable.

INNOVATIONS INCORPORATED INTO CIFFTA'S ONLINE PLATFORM

Our CIFFTA team believes strongly that innovations are needed to create evidence-based training and implementation methods, just as we needed the innovations in evidence-based family treatments described in earlier chapters. To tackle these challenges in a systematic and scientific way, we formed a company, Training and Implementation Associates (TIA). Funded by grants from the National Institute of Mental Health, we have developed and tested a platform that we feel has the potential to disrupt the training and implementation field. In the remainder of this chapter, we describe the major components that we believe can lead to improved training and implementation, how we met the challenges outlined above, and how we expanded the work to address additional challenges at the organization level of community-based treatment programs. (For access to the CIFFTA online training platform, please follow this link: *www.guilford.com/santisteban-materials.*)

Thinking Differently about What Therapists Should Be Learning

Our work began with the well-established family therapy and CIFFTA competencies we have emphasized in this book: (1) systemic conceptualization, (2) engagement of family members, (3) eliciting motivation, (4) reducing maladaptive and increasing supportive family interactions, and (5) tailoring CIFFTA to the unique characteristics and needs of families. As we moved to organize the CIFFTA competencies around subtasks that the family therapist must master, we rediscovered the usefulness of the Nelson et al. (2007) framework that moves beyond conceptual understanding and emphasizes conceptual, perceptual, and executive elements. This framework emphasizes more than just an understanding of an intervention but also the ability to recognize the clinical situation in which a specific intervention would be useful, and the ability to deliver the intervention (Nelson et al., 2007). Said differently, you not only learn what intervention you should use and why, but you also learn to detect and identify the clinical situations in which you should use the intervention, and you practice delivery of the intervention. This is the type of comprehensive training that can help you feel confident as you integrate new practices.

Dansereau and Dees (2002) emphasize how important it is for practice sessions to integrate "thinking" and "doing." They argue that didactic training tends to be linear, whereas practice is multidimensional and dynamic. Practice and discussions of practice help to integrate the "what" and the "why" and is a necessary step before the counselor feels comfortable with the new strategy or technique. As Laszloffy and Hardy (2000) have argued about addressing racism in therapy sessions, knowing that it is important to address an issue is different from becoming competent and comfortable in addressing the issue in sessions.

An Online Platform on Which to Learn and Practice CIFFTA

Our CIFFTA online training and coaching platform integrates many of the advances and opportunities we have discussed: (1) It begins with the five major CIFFTA competencies; (2) it breaks down the competencies to identify knowledge (conceptual) and skills (perceptual/seeing and execution/doing) for each competency; (3) it provides interactive videos and quizzes that ensure learning is taking place; (4) it provides 3D characters (avatars) simulating clinical situations that show the learner what a good delivery looks like; (5) it provides practice opportunities in which trainees show their skill in identifying situations and in the delivery of interventions; (6) it provides a system (used in both training and coaching) for reviewing recorded trainee practice interventions and for placing expert comments right into the recording so that trainees receive very specific feedback to each of their responses; and (7) it provides 24/7 access to the training platform and tools (e.g., treatment manual, psychoeducational modules).

A training case example may be helpful here. Below we show the use of the online platform to highlight the strengths of the CIFFTA model in teaching one of the most important interventions in family therapy: How to engage a family member who is reluctant to engage into treatment and feels coerced into treatment. As we discussed in Chapter 6, family therapy can only be successful if you can engage the family members who are reluctant to attend sessions. Remember that those reluctant family members are often the most critical pieces in the family puzzle.

In the case of Jennifer, a therapist new to family therapy, the platform begins by providing instructive information that she needs to conceptualize the nature of the engagement problem. It helps Jennifer understand the limitations of the word *resistance* and the often-understandable reasons families may have to be reluctant to engage in treatment (e.g., poor experiences with past therapists and therapy systems). Jennifer learns about the patterns that clients demonstrate around reluctance to engage in treatment; patterns based on research on engagement (Santisteban & Szapocznik, 1994; Santisteban et al., 1996). The platform demonstrates each pattern, for example, when a caregiver feels coerced into treatment by a school or a juvenile justice system and they perceive the therapist to be an ally of the system that is disempowering them. Jennifer begins to understand the importance of distinguishing her role and goals from those of the larger referring system. She learns about the importance of not being perceived as part of a system (e.g., the juvenile justice system) that punishes the youth for a transgression.

Jennifer interacts with animated caregivers communicating this reluctance to enter treatment and expressing their feeling of being coerced in direct or indirect ways. By comparing this clinical situation to other situations demonstrated by avatars (e.g., when a caregiver wants treatment but the adolescent refuses), Jennifer gains mastery in distinguishing the different patterns associated with reluctance to engage in treatment. She gets to see what a client looks like in the therapy room when they are displaying each specific pattern. We then provide simulations demonstrating how she can intervene in the different scenarios presented by the reluctant family member.

Finally, clinical simulations present an example of a caregiver who feels coerced into treatment and Jennifer is asked to respond as if she were speaking to the client in a therapy session. Our CIFFTA team of experts reviews the recorded video or audio-only response and provides specific feedback on her intervention. The feedback is provided in direct relationship to each part of the intervention she presented to the client so that the feedback is focused, clear, and useful. The expert feedback helps to shape the therapist's communication, much as the therapist attempts to shape family communications in sessions.

The core steps, in sum, include didactic presentation of the concept, case simulation to illustrate the concept, avatars to help the therapist identify patterns, demonstration of therapeutic interventions, requesting that the trainee intervene in a clinical simulation, and receiving feedback (and offering an opportunity to respond to the feedback). These steps are followed for each of the different CIFFTA platform courses on systemic conceptualization, engagement, enhancing motivation, reducing family conflict and other risk factors, and increasing family support.

Using this set of tools, strategies, and procedures, the expert team shapes the practice interventions you try and helps increase your level of effectiveness and confidence. The process of shaping specific therapist interventions is isomorphic with the process you use in shaping the interactions in the family. Rather than providing vague and overly general feedback, the best feedback shapes the communications with specificity. It is important to note that although our online training and implementation platform has initially been used with CIFFTA, it is considered "agnostic" with respect to content, meaning that it can be used to provide any training content. For example, given that motivation enhancement is part of the work we do, we have an entire course on that set of skills. Therapists familiar with MI know that using client verbalizations to identify the stages of change is a critical part of the needed *perceptual* skill set. Our ability to use avatars to teach the learner to distinguish between precontemplation and contemplation in sessions is key to knowing what to do next.

As is evident in the examples above, the innovative use of video technology is proving to be an important tool for moving the online experience from a passive process to one in which the trainee interacts with the learning platform in more "therapy-like" ways. Fine-tuning the ability to identify complex clinical processes or behaviors through the video presentation of clinical simulation and to analyze what you see (e.g., showing the skill of seeing/detecting) can be particularly important because of the complexities of family processes. For example, in CIFFTA's perceptual domain within "modifying family interactions," you assess a family interaction and detect where "things go wrong." Faced with a clinical simulation, you are asked to do the analysis and describe the family interactions using CIFFTA terminology learned in the previous lesson (e.g., expressions of support/conflict, alliances/coalitions, invalidation). You are also asked to describe (via a recording) what you perceive to be the session *content* (e.g., what is spoken about) versus what you see as *process* (e.g., the family dance and pattern of relating). The ability to distinguish process and content is a major family therapy competency. After you complete the analysis, you receive expert feedback in very practice-oriented language that suggests different ways of seeing clinical processes and/or delivering the intervention. The more you practice, the more confident you will feel when the time comes for implementation with a real family. Areas in need of further training/remediation (e.g., confusing process and content) can be addressed by adding training and ancillary resources.

In the next step of the family process example above, you demonstrate mastery of therapeutic skills or interventions (e.g., blocking a hostile family interaction) by responding to a presentation of a clinical situation. In the video response you *do,* as opposed to saying what you *would do* (e.g., recording what you would say to block or reframe a hurtful and hostile family communication). When you have little experience in blocking a person who tends to control the flow of communication, it may feel awkward, disrespectful, and even aggressive at first. With practice, you find the words and comfort to block and redirect a communication in a respectful way that you are comfortable with. Only with practice does the learner become increasingly confident that the necessary tools are now in their therapeutic toolbox.

In the following box we share another important example of how the learner interfaces with the technology, how practice is facilitated, and how expert feedback serves to shape the learner's interventions.

The example focuses on highly sensitive and complex issue (i.e., racism) because there has been much written on how a therapist can understand the importance of addressing such a sensitive issue but still feel incapable of comfortably addressing it (Laszloffy & Hardy, 2000). When the therapist does not feel that they can address the issue in an effective way, it will be avoided, and this avoidance will inevitably be perceived by the client and will damage the therapeutic relationship. With practice and expert feedback, the therapist can become increasingly comfortable with ways of validating and evoking more from the client related to the experience.

> ### A Trainee's Experience on the Training Platform
>
> - *Youth client avatar (seen by therapist in-training):* "Teachers at that school are racist. If a Black or Hispanic kid argues, they suspend them immediately. But then other kids can go farther and even get into fights, and they don't get suspended."
>
> - *Therapist avatar (seen by therapist-in-training):* "It is not uncommon to run into racist folks and even systems. Tell me more about how you feel racism impacts your well-being and success at school."
>
> - *Therapist-in-training is asked to respond to the animation (in a recording):* "The above example is a simulation of a contextual influence impacting the youth and family. Please provide a recording of what you would say to this youth and consider how the family can be brought into the solution. Please say it exactly as you would say it to the client/family."
>
> - *Example of a therapist-in-training's recorded response submitted to the platform:* "I hear you. Racism is very real, and it is normal to feel angry when you feel that people who look like you are being treated unfairly. Tell me more about your experience and how it has made you feel so far."
>
> - *Expert feedback received by the therapist—feedback typed right into the recording:* "You did well validating the client and normalizing their experience with racism. You also elicited the client's experience by asking that he share more. You can also check in with the client to see if they have ever talked about this with their family. To fully utilize the family as a resource, you might say something like 'Given everything going on at the school and how it has affected you, what do you think about talking more about this during a family session and discussing ways in which to make your voice heard in a healthy and effec-

> tive way? Your family has lots of experience with this type of stressor and how institutions respond when the issue is raised.'"
>
> ---
>
> You can find out more about TIA International's innovative training platform at *www.guilford.com/santisteban-materials*. There you can see a demonstration of how the system works and explore TIA's resources and products.

Improved Standardization and Tailoring of Content

There are added benefits and advantages to the type of platform that we have developed. The first is the standardization of training content and processes. Within this system, users receive the same content consistently and there is less concern that the therapy content will vary from training to training. Of course, the fact that the content is in a central location also allows it to be updated and enhanced more easily. The same is true for training processes that may vary from trainer to trainer and from event to event. Material or exercises are not skipped or modified in a way that affect the impact of the course and fidelity to the original treatment.

A second advantage is that the platform can more easily be tailored to the needs of the learner. The system is adaptive in that additional learning material, examples, animations/simulations, and practice exercises can be made available to a learner in the specific areas they are struggling with. Large-group training events typically keep on moving in a preset direction regardless of the speed of knowledge acquisition of the learners. A third advantage is that the system can be adapted to client preferences by moving from the more typical asynchronous learning activities to synchronous activities. The traditional eLearning is asynchronous, with no predetermined time for the learning to take place. Everyone can go at their own pace and take their time to learn what they need to know, when they need to know it. However, more synchronous eLearning that occurs in real-time or simultaneously can also be offered through web conferencing and chat options if that is preferred.

Using an adaptive framework for coaching allows that work to be tailored just as it is tailored during the initial training phase. Implementation challenges become most visible once implementation with real clients has started, and skills must be practiced. At this point the coach has more specific feedback to provide. As noted previously, ongoing supervision and support have been found to be critical factors in the success of training implementation and long-term sustainability.

Our platform is an example of how coaching can be used in innovative ways. Because we use various methods to assess trainees' knowledge and skills during training, the trainee profile allows trainers, coaches, or supervisors to monitor progress and tailor coaching based on individual strengths and weaknesses. Under this model, coaches not only expand the knowledge and skills taught in training, but they also impart craft knowledge (e.g., engagement, ethics, managing workflow, clinical judgment). Like the approach taken in the trainee practice videos, the coach can place comments right onto the recording of a therapy session, so that the trainee has feedback specific to each word or phrase they used or feedback on a family process they may have missed (e.g., how an adolescent shuts down when certain conversations take a specific tone). This coaching tool shapes the therapist's communication in a highly precise way. Another valuable aspect of this coaching process is its ease of use. This is all done online at whatever time is convenient for the coach and the trainee. This is a significant improvement over the traditional method of having to schedule in-person sessions to review a video.

Creating Community Using a Peer Learning Network

As noted earlier in the chapter, one challenge to online platforms is the perceived loss of community. The effectiveness of connecting clinicians with peers and trainers has been documented in the field of behavioral health (Nadeem et al., 2013). In situations such as web-based training where face-to-face contact with trainers and peers is more limited, the interaction of peers in a group setting can be accomplished through a professional learning community or a peer learning network (PLN). In our work we have begun to use virtual PLN meetings to support ongoing use of effective practices and create a sense of community. It is sometimes also helpful to create a forum where participants can post questions and resources between coaching and/or PLN meetings.

The PLN has the added benefit that it encourages members to take ownership of their community and to share knowledge and successful implementation strategies. Following the Markiewicz et al. (2006) Learning Collaborative Toolkit Model, we have used PLN to focus on adopting best practices in diverse service settings; enacting interactive training methods, and skill-focused learning; adapting effective practices to their settings; and capitalizing on shared learning and collaboration. Examples of topics discussed by our PLN participants include (1) learning how to identify strengths in families and mobilize protective factors; (2) identifying how cultural factors impact how families define and label problems, how they ask for help, and their likelihood of engaging in services; (3) cultural and societal implications on LGBTQ+ mental health and well-being; (4) the impact of immigration, intergenerational trauma, and separations on families; (5) identifying and discussing systemic and structural inequities; and (6) treating families and adolescents with trauma.

Improving Implementation and Sustainment at Community Treatment Agencies

Over decades, our work with highly committed treatment agencies who seek to develop their workforce has demonstrated that bringing evidence-based family therapy to the forefront of practice and maintaining its implementation with a high level of fidelity has proven to be difficult. Many have argued that the investment in training has not translated into an institutional capacity to maintain high-quality services in community settings (Novins et al., 2013). The everyday practice of EBTs is not very well sustained after initial implementation (Stirman et al., 2012). This may be particularly true for family therapy, which comes with additional challenges in terms of working with multiple family members and juggling multiple alliances. Organizations that are now beyond the "Does family therapy work?" question are ripe for innovations that meet the unique challenges that family therapy pose, the organizational challenges that agencies face as they seek to adopt and implement family therapy, and the innovations that can propel the field forward. Organizational factors such as supervision, monitoring, leadership, and allocation of resources must be mobilized and aligned to achieve practice level quality and fidelity (Beidas & Kendall 2010; Fixsen et al., 2005).

Unfortunately, factors found to be critical for sustainment at the agency level are not typically part of traditional training strategies and plans. Randell (2012) sees organizational culture and staffing as particularly thorny challenges. To optimize sustainability of EBTs, we must help organizations assess their readiness to accept the change that evidence-based practices demand. Continuous monitoring and adjustments are essential for effective management of EBTs. With respect to staffing, we must be prepared to work with therapists accustomed to high levels of autonomy in their practice and not used to higher levels of monitoring. According to Randell (2012) there are key questions that can be asked: Has the EBT become an established way of doing business? Is there a specific pattern of resistance to adoption? Were the foundations for change successfully laid at the outset of the EBT initiative? Furthermore, compounding questions regarding model fidelity and general sustainability are presented: Are there enough clinicians certified to deliver the service? Can the agency retain them once trained? We must also ask whether supervisors are trained well enough to guide the supervisees on the new EBT.

A closer look at the changes asked of therapists is helpful here.

Therapists in community settings often work with large caseloads of clients, and they cannot control the size of their caseload as can be done in private settings. The new therapy may be based on assumptions different from their own about what therapy should attempt to change. Transitioning away from the therapy model in which they were originally trained takes extra energy and effort. Oliver and Lang (2018) found that competing demands for time impede implementation for most community agencies. Even when clinicians embrace the new EBT, they may run into the reality of an agency that is not fully supportive of the requirements of sustaining the new practice. These sustainability requirements may include the need for additional coaching or supervision, additional time to complete fidelity and outcome measures, and video recording of sessions to facilitate coaching processes and ensure fidelity.

For an agency, perhaps the most challenging aspect of sustaining an EBT with fidelity is staff turnover. Staff turnover eliminates the benefits of recent training efforts and directly disrupts sustainability. Aaron et al. (2009) suggest that turnover becomes more likely when staff go through the stress of learning a new EBT without the necessary support and coaching to help them master the new practice. Some staffing disruptions come not from people leaving the agency but from internal promotions that moved an EBT champion or leader to a different department or unit.

Agency Readiness Work to Address Organizational Culture and Practices

Culturally, organizations must assess their readiness to accept the change that evidence-based practices demand, with some organizations having to challenge ingrained attitudes and practices. The questions about organizational culture and implications for implementation and sustainability also point to the work that needs to be done with clinicians. Clinicians in community settings are often experienced, and they are already committed to a particular therapy model. The task of integrating competing models is not an easy one. Even when clinicians embrace the new EBT, they may run into the reality of an agency that is not prepared to support the requirements of sustaining the new practice (e.g., additional coaching or supervision, additional time completing fidelity and outcome measures, video recording of sessions to ensure fidelity).

We emphasize the importance of identifying and engaging the organization's "champions" for that new EBT to help promote the treatment with their staff and maintain the needed level of commitment and resources throughout the training, coaching, and implementation stages. In our work we recommend an agency readiness and implementation consultation designed to assess organizational factors and the identification and engagement of the organization's *champions*. EBT champions work with their teams to promote adoption and practice and maintain a high level of commitment throughout the training, coaching, and implementation stages. Our agency readiness work includes (1) online assessment of agency readiness; (2) online meetings with the leaders and clinical supervisors to present the results of the readiness assessment process and discuss the implications for training and implementation; and (3) follow-up online meetings with the leaders of each agency and/or clinical supervisors to discuss any modifications that may be needed before the start of the project.

In our work with agencies, we focus on supervisor training as an essential component of our approach. The supervisor training is an adaptation of the counselor training and includes conceptualization of the case, strategies to tailor the engagement and interventions, and discussion of techniques used in the delivery of each component. By reviewing recorded sessions, we utilize fidelity ratings to measure competence in key areas and to direct the tailoring of the consultation, which may include viewing live or recorded sessions.

Addressing Disruptions Resulting from Staff Turnover

Agencies are constantly promoting staff, transferring them to a different position or unit, or losing employees who join a different organization. Inviting an EBT expert to travel across the country for a 2- to 3-day in-person training event is not a practical way to train a highly fluid workforce. Often, the unspoken solution to training new staff is to have previously trained staff do the training, even if they are not equipped to do so. This introduces significant variation in the training experiences of different staff. By using an online learning platform that has been proven effective in training staff, the new staff training process can start on day one without any delays. The training is standardized so that there is no drift or watering down process with each subsequent training. Achieving the right balance between training and ongoing coaching and support is critically important because studies have reported that staff turnover may in fact be worsened during the early stages of EBT implementation, if the right support is not provided (Randell, 2012). Without dedicated and readily accessible internal support, this work can be overwhelmingly stressful and can increase turnover (Aarons et al., 2009). This is certainly not a result that agencies had counted on. If the initial exposure and training can occur in a more cost-effective manner, there can be more attention and resources allocated to support, consultation, and sustaining the type of therapy that can help clients.

Our agency consultation helps leaders better understand how an overemphasis on multiple exposure/training experiences with varied treatments neglects the importance of ongoing support, coaching, and EBT-specific supervision. One specific example of the need for coaching and consultation is when there is a need for cultural adaptation in the delivery of the EBT. This occurs when an EBT is used with clients of diverse races and ethnicities and who experience unique stressors and life experiences not addressed by mainstream EBTs. In these situations, coaching sessions can provide the support and guidance on EBT adaptations, and this can relieve the stress on therapists.

An example serves to illustrate how online training can contribute to keeping a fluid workforce well-trained. On a project in which we were contracted to deliver online CIFFTA training and to secure in-person training for a separate EBT that has an excellent network of trainers, the differences in handling staff turnover were dramatic. Over a two-year span there was a 40% turnover rate in the five sites that were participating in the project. Sites delivering the online CIFFTA had immediate access to training for newly hired staff. For the sites doing in-person training, it took months to get new staff trained. The systemic turnover conditions made it difficult to keep up, especially when turnover occurred soon after completion of an in-person training event. It is important to point out that this experience is not specific to any intervention.

Maintaining Fidelity

Another important factor in sustainability is the need for effective and efficient methods to monitor and enhance fidelity. To achieve the best possible outcomes, practitioners of an EBT must follow the prescribed guidelines and procedures. Our online platform increases the consistency of implementation by standardizing the training and coaching procedures into a uniform package that can be revisited as part of a refresher plan. This comprehensive approach to standardization of training and implementation makes it less susceptible to the "drifting" that usually takes place over time. We also provide tools that help the practitioner keep a focus on fidelity (e.g., self-rating fidelity tool).

Fiscal Considerations

One of the constraints which is often overlooked in EBT sustainability is financial costs. Aarons et al. (2009) found that cost was the most important and least changeable factor in EBT implementation. An often-overlooked aspect of live training is that it requires that staff attend in groups, thus removing staff from their important and revenue-generating functions. Time and financial pressures faced by those charged with bringing the interventions into their settings (e.g., agency leaders) can lead to attempts to manage costs. In the absence of data on the most effective way to learn and master competencies, there will be varied attempts to reduce training and coaching hours. Implementation shortcuts often lead to a potential loss of benefit (McHugh & Barlow, 2010).

Online training seeks to address these problems in a couple of major ways. First, staff do not have to participate in groups, so the flexibility of scheduling is increased. Second, the training is available at any time, including times when there is less client contact and clinical responsibilities. Trainees can schedule the training themselves, during their "slowest" hours, instead of their high-demand hours. Finally, recognizing cost as an important factor in sustainability, we have made our platform more cost-effective through such factors as the use of animation instead of actors, the use of digital voices as opposed to human voice-overs, and by incorporating elements like eLearning-enhanced instructional design techniques.

Reducing the cost of the initial training is most beneficial if it can allow for a more tailored training and implementation process that can help narrow the longstanding research-to-practice gap. A more cost-effective solution can help agencies that are unable to afford the ongoing and high costs for training and consultation and that end up purchasing only the orientation and face-to-face training visits (which do not lead to competence in a new and complex EBT). The ability of online platforms to deliver cost-efficient training and coaching means that they could be of great benefit to agencies that would otherwise have to forgo successful implementation of EBTs. This is especially important for those agencies with limited resources, and which often tend to provide services to large, underserved populations.

Additional Challenges That Organizations Must Address

As the field of EBT implementation and online platforms matures, there are additional challenges that have emerged. One of the issues that agencies are currently dealing with is that when therapists are certified as competent in an EBT, it makes them more marketable and may increase the likelihood that they leave the agency for higher salaries. EBT certification may have the unintended consequence of contributing to turnover. One new idea is to certify agencies rather than trainees; agencies are, after all, the ones investing capital in training. This also reflects the fact that the agency is making an investment by providing the necessary support needed for sustainment (e.g., smaller caseloads, supervisors, and champions). Other agencies are trying to address this problem by requesting a contractual commitment from new clinical hires.

Coaching and consultation can benefit from having recorded sessions to review but therapists often have concerns about recordings that EBTs require as part of the practitioner training and EBT program fidelity monitoring. Given that recordings and the associated technical requirements cause problems for a surprising number of organizations, providers should make the effort to integrate the recording process with the clinical environment, minimizing the distractions whenever possible. Agencies must reassure their clients with secured, state-of-the-science technology that allows for secure communications and online consultation of family cases, including live therapy sessions (thus avoiding the issue of permanent recordings). The networking environment must give special consideration to ethical standards and be fully compliant with the Health Insurance Portability and Accountability Act (HIPAA).

CONTINUOUS RESEARCH TO IMPROVE TRAINING, IMPLEMENTATION, AND SUSTAINABILITY

Consistent with this call for action, TIA is conducting rigorous research to investigate how well our platform can work to overcome these challenges. An online platform must not only deliver the training more efficiently and with high acceptance, but it must also show that it is not inferior to the traditional in-person training with respect to the trainee's mastery of the competencies. The preliminary research on our online platform has shown that it is equivalent or slightly better than an in-person comparison condition in producing significant improvement in family therapy competencies (Santisteban et al., 2024) and we are currently conducting a full randomized trial funded by the National Institute of Mental Health to provide a more rigorous test.

SUMMARY AND ONGOING CHALLENGES

In this chapter, we argue that not all training efforts are created equal and that having an EBT does not guarantee its adoption and sustainability in the field. The time is right for designing and testing evidence-based and cost-effective methods for training and implementation that can address longstanding challenges at the level of the individual therapist who wishes to learn family therapy. The same is true at the level of leadership in service organizations that strive to improve their workforce by training them in addressing the needs of families using evidence-based family therapy. In this chapter we reviewed the challenges pertaining to the *training and mastery* of a new EBT at the individual practitioner level and the challenges pertaining to *implementation and sustainment* of EBTs at the agency level.

For each of the major challenges, we showed how technical innovations can positively impact the field and how our CIFFTA online training platform has attempted to incorporate these advances. With a focus on the promise of technology and online platforms, we showed how novel implementation activities can address the challenges to training and mastery. The application of our online platform demonstrates how bringing together these advances in technology (e.g., online training, simulation, interactive videos), new ways of conceptualizing and isolating family therapy competencies, and proven strategies for increasing treatment agency readiness, may represent a disruptive movement that can change the way family therapy skills are taught, mastered, and sustained. Simulation training is cost-effective and instructionally effective for professional development. We will continue to promote research to ensure that we create evidence-based training and implementation practices that are worthy of the EBTs we seek to provide in all communities. If we can succeed with such a platform, this training also lends itself to translation into other languages and thus broader dissemination internationally.

10

Extensions to New Populations, Unique Applications, and Future Directions for CIFFTA

In this chapter we share how CIFFTA is being used in non-Latine populations, in unique clinical circumstances, and we talk about the enhancements we have planned for future work. CIFFTA was originally developed to address stressors experienced by Latine families (Mena et al., 2008b; Santisteban, 2013). Throughout its development, we sought to ensure that the voices and experiences of these families were used to refine and enhance the treatment. This meant using culture-related information to guide the mobilization of protection in the face of often-unsupportive environments. We believe CIFFTA created a template that is well equipped for helping other diverse and marginalized populations.

The Minority Stress Model introduced in Chapter 2 (Meyer, 2003; Goldbach & Gibbs, 2015) is a helpful framework for working with other non-Latine minoritized and marginalized populations. We define Minority Stress as the excess stress to which individuals from stigmatized social categories are exposed as a result of their social, often minoritized position. These stressors can include discrete events or chronic and long-standing conditions related to social structures and policies that fail to support all people equally. For example, there are systemic and structural inequities that negatively impact Black families and part of our work must be to better identify and name these systemic and structural inequities. Too often these influences are conflated with cultural factors, but they are outside of the client and the client's culture (Wilcox, 2023). Being distrustful and/or angry are not part of a cultural worldview but are predictable consequences of racism and anti-immigrant sentiment. Therefore, when developing strategies and techniques for helping people who are oppressed in this way, we must learn to recognize and effectively integrate these topics into therapy. We must be totally cognizant that certain systems and structures have historically led to detrimental impacts on the mental health of some clients (Wilcox, 2023). Supporters of a Liberatory Psychology approach (Burton & Guzzo, 2020) emphasize the importance of highlighting and reinforcing cultural strengths and resilience in the face of oppressive conditions. Clinicians need to become adept at not only understanding oppressive conditions and influences on clients' lived experiences, but to detect them, make them increasingly visible, and integrate them into a systemic conceptualization and treatment plan. In CIFFTA, we are working to ensure that therapists are trained to go beyond developing *racial awareness,* the understanding of effects of racism. We aim to develop racial sensitivity by equipping therapists with the skills to seamlessly integrate this understanding into the evaluation and treatment of clients' presenting problems, ensuring that clients feel truly understood. (Laszloffy & Hardy, 2000). Clinicians must become comfortable exploring topics of discrimination that can be communicated directly or indirectly by clients. By naming it, you create a space for acknowledging the effects of discrimination on clients, families, and presenting concerns. As we noted in Laszloffy and Hardy's work (2000), knowing what you should do does not mean you can identify the moments when your intervention is needed and does not mean you have practiced the delivery of sensitive messages so that you can comfortably and confidently use them.

The minority stress framework can help the provider to identify, comfortably discuss, and validate the experiences of diverse clients. This is a first step toward fully engaging a client and creating a tailored treatment plan that promotes resilience in those stressful contexts. The minority stress model reminds us to include a focus on both the *distal* stressors that exist outside the individual such as stereotypes, discrimination, and prejudice as well as the *proximal* stressors that are more internalized reactions and responses that come from being chronically exposed to these harmful messages. Many of the clients we describe in this chapter have experienced minority stress and all the additional stressors that come with belonging to a group that is seen as "other" and whose culture-related diversity are not always affirmed and validated by policies and structures.

EXTENDING CIFFTA TO NON-LATINE POPULATIONS

In this section we provide examples of the way in which CIFFTA's culturally informed template is extended to include material that is particularly relevant and timely for different communities we have served.

Using CIFFTA to Work with Haitian Youth and Families

Haitian youth and families have migrated in large numbers to the South Florida area in search of more opportunity, safety from political turmoil and violence, and in the hopes that their children can have a brighter future. As with most immigrant families, the journey to that bright future is often difficult and the unwelcoming reception that some families receive in the larger community can make that journey particularly treacherous and damaging.

The CIFFTA team was fortunate to partner with a team from the Department of Anthropology at the University of Miami that conducted ethnographic research and sought to use that knowledge to better serve the community (Cela et al., 2023). They chose to use the CIFFTA template of culturally informed youth and family services to treat youth who were engaging in substance use or at risk for substance use and who were mandated to treatment within the local Juvenile Services Department's (JSD's) prevention and diversion programs. The treatment development project was funded by the National Institute on Drug Abuse. As part of this work, Cela et al. (2023) published on the experiences of youth and families, in their own voices, as they experience structural racism and socioethnic discrimination. The work describes in detail the ways in which adolescents become increasingly aware of racism and discrimination in a school system, and in a "justice" system that does not always treat all youth equitably based on the same problem behaviors.

A difficult and complex situation arose in the treatment teams as they attempted to provide quality care to youth who have been offered diversion programs and alternatives to arrest, because they realized that many of the youth should not be in the system. This conclusion is clear when one compares the consequences suffered by low-income Haitian youth in comparison to other youth and families with enough resources to hire a lawyer who can keep them out of the system despite even worse offenses. The stress experienced by therapists who try to do important work despite feeling they are part of a system that is responding unjustly, is a stress that must be investigated in the field and that may require additional support for the team.

Immigration-Related Stressors

In working with recent immigrants, the therapist encounters a great sense of loss, disorientation, despair, and loss of support and identity. Recent immigrants may also lose occupational status when they cannot use the professional degree they had in their country of origin or must take on jobs that are at a much lower rung in terms of pay and/or status. There are a multitude of contextual factors that can impact the well-being of the immigrant including reception in the host community and neighborhood, density of immigrants in the neighborhood, and varied socioeconomic factors (Abraído-Lanza et al., 2016).

Cervantes and colleagues have been among the field's leaders in identifying and systematically measuring the types and severity of stressors related not only to acculturation but also to being a recent immigrant (see Chapter 2). Because families leave their countries of origin for varied reasons, it is important for therapists to identify the life experiences that led them to leave their country (e.g., war, famine, persecution, desire for upward mobility) and the continuing impact of these experiences on their daily lives. The path to the United States can also be traumatic for families who had a dangerous and perilous journey. It is common for family members to suffer in silence and feel it is not worth discussing the painful events. The traumatic conditions they fled, and the immigration and acculturation processes can all have powerful and negative impacts on family systems and family functioning.

The postmigration period is particularly difficult for families whose arrival is not formally sanctioned. Among the factors identified in this type of research are fear of deportation and exposure to trauma during migration (Cervantes et al., 2018). Once here, families who are undocumented or do not have formal permission to be in the United States cannot avail themselves of all the services and support that is typically provided to families in need. For example, victims of domestic violence may feel unable to report the violence for fear that they or the perpetrator may be deported. Similarly, illegal or "delinquent" behavior by a youth must be kept secret for fear of disproportionate repercussions including deportation. In this way, social and concrete support that is designed to help strengthen families, may be avoided by the fearful client. In short, the fear of being identified and deported means undocumented families must stay as hidden and invisible as possible.

Acculturation Processes and Their Impact on the Family

Acculturation-related process have a powerful impact on Haitian family relationships. Some are like those encountered with Latine families and that originally led to the cultural adaptations that are part of CIFFTA. These include the fact that Haitian families often embrace hierarchy, strict obedience on the part of children, strong family discipline, and respect for traditional principles that regulate family relations in Haiti. Acculturation implies internalization of different values including an ethos of egalitarianism and individualism. When the principle of hierarchy is threatened, family functioning can become maladaptive. Families may feel that the *American* culture and the therapies that derive from them are misguided and overly permissive. This is a common theme in work with Haitian families. The growing discrepancy between parents who acculturate much more slowly and youth who acculturate very rapidly, can exacerbate existing generational differences and conflicts and lead to considerable family breakdowns (Santisteban et al., 2013). Treatment must focus on all these culture-related dynamics and their impacts on the family. Therapy must start by normalizing the within-family acculturation discrepancies and the within-family tensions they generate. It is also important to avoid prematurely challenging the hierarchy—for example, by encouraging the adolescent to share their perspectives and needs or by insinuating to families early on that this is not the way things work in the United States. This would be incongruent with the worldview of many Haitian parents who value respect, authority, and obedience (Clermont-Mathieu & Nicolas, 2016).

An important component of therapy is to facilitate an ecological perspective that considers the impact of all the systems that touch the youth and family. This framework helps caregivers think about how to become better advocates for their youth in school, health, legal, and other systems. The therapist must also appreciate, however, that there may be culture-related worldviews and perspectives that make engagement of these institutions and systems more difficult (Santisteban et al., 2013). Besides language barriers and a severe shortage of creole-speaking counselors and school staff, Haitian families may have a worldview that engenders respect and deference for large institutions, which in turn makes families less likely to try to challenge the system and advocate for their youth. Marcelin (2012) points out that Haitian families may have a unique perspective on the role of government in the private lives of individuals, which reduces the likelihood that they would seek to challenge these systems. This may be in part due to a fear of law enforcement, but it also comes from a broader set of cultural beliefs. In the work by the therapy team mentioned at the start of this section, this meant that parents were less likely to challenge institutions (e.g., school, legal) that may have been displaying behavior that could be called discriminatory. Marcelin (2012) reports that parents who have lived in Haiti are not used to institutions that set rules for private life (e.g., compulsory schooling, defining child abuse and domestic violence) and that for these reasons parents find themselves in unfamiliar, uncomfortable, and intimidating territory. One can imagine how this unfamiliar pattern of government involvement in personal life can lead to resentment and the feeling of being disempowered by powerful systems. Families that are thrown off balance by this reality may feel helpless and hopeless and less likely to engage in family treatment. Haitian parents' apprehension of government agencies stems from a sociopolitical history of oppression, corruption, and violence in their home country as well as fear of persecution by U.S. immigration officials because of their unresolved immigration status. This mistrust has also extended to schools and other social service agencies. Clermont-Mathieu and Nicolas (2016) describe the strong value in Haitian families that endorses concealing the disappointments and failures of the family from the outside world. This helps the therapist to understand how painful it is when a youngster's behavior brings attention and outside monitoring to the family. In treatment it is helpful to use psychoeducation to help the family process this stigma and shame, and to help them understand key institutions, including the juvenile justice system, and how to best interact with their different representatives (e.g., public defenders and probation officers).

Even for families who are documented and have access to all the needed services, there may be values and worldviews that make it difficult to interact effectively with important systems in the community. Hofstede's (1980) concept of Power Distance explains why many newcomers to the United States believe that formal institutions (e.g., juvenile justice system and schools) must be treated with profound respect, conformity, and deference. Programs that include multisystemic interventions designed to encourage parents to become strong advocates for the well-being of the youth must understand when the interventions are going against the cultural norms. It takes clinical skill to work through the discrepancy. It is also important to avoid erroneously labeling parents as overly passive, dependent, and lacking in motivation when the hesitation comes from a cultural belief or value. Work that focuses on the interactions between recent immigrants and large institutions would do well to consider the influence of Hofstede's power distance orientation in their work.

At times, and to be extremely careful with the well-being of the youth, parents attempt to prohibit youth from spending time outside the home with friends who can create risky situations and lead to the triggering of government involvement. This protection is especially true when parents feel their peers do not share the same family values (Clermont-Mathieu & Nicolas, 2016). Unfortunately, this position can become extreme, can deny the youth the opportunity to socialize and grow in their individuality, and can lead youth to rebel against parental authority. This is often the foundation of further family breakdown and is a key area in which we can see the benefits of family therapy.

Our Haitian colleagues from anthropology have pointed to additional realities in the lives of the local Haitian community that could impact their well-being and the work of a therapist. First, they point out that coming from one of the poorest countries in the world, many Haitian immigrants in south Florida lack the education and financial wherewithal through which other immigrant groups have benefitted in establishing themselves in the host country. For clients who are undereducated and with low literacy in both English and their native language, this means adjusting the psychoeducational modules so that they are easily understood and utilized.

Furthermore, stigma related to mental health and lack of context for therapeutic services also contribute to disparities in seeking and receiving treatment among minority groups. Haitians adjusting to a new cultural context may be accustomed to seeking treatment from outside a formal health care system and lack trust, or confidence that care will be congruent with their cultural values (Rastogi et al., 2012). As presented in Chapter 2, many recent immigrants will be planning for or going through a reunification following a youth and family separation and this is a process that can be effectively addressed in family therapy (Mitrani et al., 2004; Suárez-Orozco & Suárez-Orozco, 2001).

Using CIFFTA to Work with African American and Other Black Youth and Families

In extending CIFFTA to work with African American and other Black youth, one area that has recently emerged as concerning is self-harm among Black youth. In the period leading up to 2017, there was a dramatic rise in self-harm behaviors in Black youth and in the prevalence of suicide attempts (Kann et al., 2018). Price and Khubchandani (2019) reported that "the rate of African American male suicides increased by 60% and for African American female suicides increased by 182% from 2001 to 2017" (p. 756). These alarming trends have led to a congressional task force report highlighting the problem, possible contributing factors, and the need for the development of services that can address the unique stressors experienced by Black youth and families (Coleman et al., 2019).

Unlike most Haitian families we work with, African American families and other Black families who have lived in the United States for generations are not immigrants trying to better understand a new system and society. They have spent all their lives identifying and dealing with a multitude of ways in which racism impacts daily life. An earlier government report highlighted how discrimination and racism damage emotional well-being through (1) internalization of negative racial stereotypes and harm to self-concept; (2) the adverse impact of chronic stressors such as living in poverty also resulting from limited opportunities due to racism; and (3) the adverse health effects resulting from daily encounters with discrimination and racism (U.S. Department of Health and Human Services, 2001). Among other social determinants of health in African American youth are high rates of incarceration, school dropout, social and economic disadvantage, and being victims of crime (Wadsworth et al., 2014). Because religious involvement is viewed as a protective factor that reduces negative outcomes in Black youth, the trend toward decreased religious involvement has also been hypothesized as a contributing factor to self-harm (Joe et al., 2007).

African American and Haitian youth and families share the fact that they encounter severe racism from many sectors of society, even including from other Black individuals from other ethnicities, which further marginalize and isolate them. This means that discussion of racism and discrimination must be multifaceted, including how to deal with injury from people that they did not expect to be marginalized by, and discussing the ways in which families can help buffer adolescents from negative consequences. The goal is that parents validate the adolescent experience and guide/lead their children on how to handle discrimination in an adaptive way.

Due to structural racism, many Black families live in communities with inadequate housing, poor educational and employment opportunities, neighborhood violence, and other social problems. This must be acknowledged in family therapy and particularly during discussions around parenting. In these types of surroundings, it means that parents must be that much more intentional and effective if they are going to succeed at buffering the youth from the high-risk factors around them. The level of parental *control* that leads to reduced behavior problems in youth varies by surroundings and parents will often feel validated when they are told that they must almost be "super-parents" to buffer their kids from risky environments (Mason et al., 1996).

Family Functioning and Protection against the Impact of Racism

In the face of such chronic and institutionalized racism, families must take on the important task of racial socialization (Jones & Neblett, 2016). This involves preparing a youth for life in a potentially unjust society, sharing survival strategies that will keep the youth safe, offering to always validate and support the youth as they confront this complex life, and instilling knowledge of, and pride in, the youth's ethnicity and race. Of course, optimal family functioning is not always present, and this complex work will be derailed by any existing family conflict and limited resources (e.g., highly overburdened families). Furthermore, because adults are not exempt from the same adverse impacts of racism and discrimination, these adverse effects may reduce the ability of families to *lead* effectively. The role of the family therapist becomes to create a space in which these painful experiences can be discussed, to validate and support the targets of racism and anti-immigrant messages, and to work to identify and enhance all the strengths that exist in that family. A culturally informed treatment is needed because it sets the expectation that these topics and this content must be present in therapy sessions if the therapy is to be considered *real, ecologically valid* (Bernal & Scharron-del Rio, 2001) and *relevant* to the lives of Black youth and families.

From the start of family therapy, the therapist must show their expertise in engaging family members, building trust, and creating a solid working relationship (Santisteban & Szapocznik, 1994). Engagement of all family members into therapy is always a complex endeavor but when working with individuals who experience the chronic stressors of racism and discrimination, it should not be surprising that there may be an added level of guardedness and remnants of distrust (Gamble, 1993). Distrust is a response to prejudice in society and should not be mistaken for characteristics of the person's culture. These should be understood for what they are, natural and expected reactions to overt or covert historical and current acts of discrimination.

Therapists must be prepared to acknowledge and openly discuss the fact that too many sectors of our society continue to judge people based on the way they say certain words, or on their foreign accents, on recent history of migration, and particularly based on skin color. The chronic stress of prejudice, discrimination, and racism is one that undermines the physical and emotional well-being of the individuals and families. The idea of racism-related stress (Harrell, 2000) and the minority stress model can be particularly useful in conceptualizing and contextualizing the presenting problems that bring Black youth and families to treatment. In addition to the *distal* factors that we have been describing above (those contextual and environmental processes that include racism), we must consider the *proximal* factors that can be interjections of the destructive outside messages based on race.

Showing an understanding of systemic forms of racism and a *willingness and ability to discuss these difficult topics* is essential when working with Black families. Too many therapists fail to understand white privilege, to understand that trust must be earned, and that an open and frank discussion about the ways in which racism impact all aspects of life is indispensable. The biggest mistake that can be made by a therapist working with Black families is to prematurely discard the idea that race and racism contributes significantly to a presenting problem. Or to believe that if race is important, the family will bring it up themselves. The fact is that it is quite common for African American families to be silent on the topics of race and racism. This occurs largely because the topic is often dismissed and invalidated by individuals and yes, even therapists, who continue to struggle with acknowledging the truth of the tentacles of racism and its current forms (Watson, 2019).

Laszloffy and Hardy (2000) articulate the subtle and not so subtle ways in which the therapist may miss opportunities to be helpful and may stumble into ways in which racism can be perpetuated in the therapy room. Racial sensitivity is needed for the therapist to actively challenge and confront the many forms racism can take. Sensitivity, of course, is not an all or nothing characteristic. The level of racial sensitivity of a therapist will influence the comfort and ease with which a therapist can discuss issues of race as part of the therapy process. One of the reasons CIFFTA seeks to build this content directly into the manualized treatment and into its training material is because it can facilitate the transfer of ideas and concepts into action. Training must focus on the ways in which therapists can turn awareness and good ideas into effective actions in the therapy room.

CIFFTA follows the wise and practical "dos and don'ts" outlined by Watson (2019) for therapists as they move toward working effectively and honestly with African American and other Black families. Although we do not list them fully here, they have much to do with understanding Whiteness and White privilege in its overt and subtle forms, feeling an obligation to not only avoid but help dismantle racist traditions and processes, being fully human and sincere in your work, and being knowledgeable and honest about history and the truths that are an integral part of our society. Within CIFFTA's work with African American and other Black families, these messages are delivered in different ways throughout all CIFFTA's components.

Jones and Neblett (2017) point out that African American youth are, according to rates of psychopathology, doing better than would be expected given the adverse conditions they often live in. They make this argument as a way of emphasizing the importance and power of resilience in this population. It is often easy to look at risk factors and problem behaviors and miss the many factors that protect youth even when faced with risky environments. At the individual level, one can enhance and strengthen racial identity. This includes helping the youth to better understand themselves, understanding how others view them, and gaining a deeper sense of pride about belonging to this race and culture. This has been shown to have a powerful buffering effect in the face of chronic stressors.

On the family side, one of the powerful resiliency factors is racial socialization. This can include sharing values, beliefs, and pride in belonging to that family and its history. In the case of Black families, racial socialization involves many forms of conveying to the youth what it means to be Black in our country, state, and community and teaching the youth strategies for effectively coping with the chronic stressor of racial discrimination.

EXTENDING CIFFTA TO WORK WITH IMPORTANT PARTNERS IN THE COMMUNITY

At times, our clinical situations have caused us to stretch and expand our thinking about the nature of the treatment team and how a truly systemic perspective allows us to do better work by integrating partners. As has been the case in our work with Latine families, our work with Haitian and African American families has benefited from the use of a Natural Helper and Community Health Worker framework. These key partners help bridge the gap between treatment services and an underserved community that has been traumatized and does not fully trust the systems around them. Community health workers often come from the community they serve and are trusted by families who are typically weary of acknowledging struggles, receiving services, or interacting in any way that makes them visible. By integrating teams of assessors and therapists with the community agency that includes the community health workers and natural helpers, we can reduce barriers to service utilization. In building the partnership the therapy team learns a great deal about the reasons and ways to get around powerful barriers and the community health workers learn a great deal about how to identify problems and how services can be helpful. Once the Community Health Worker or Natural Helper trusts the services and service providers, it becomes much easier for the family to trust the services. Engagement and retention are greatly enhanced when collaborating with these important partners.

Another key part of our experience with CIFFTA has been its use with severe substance use and chronic suicide-related and self-harm behavior that caused them to receive services from different teams in the community (Santisteban et al., 2015). In working with youth with severe symptomatology, we documented the high dosage of intensive residential treatment often needed by these youth. Whether it was hospitalizations for self-harm or residential treatment for substance use, there was a powerful need to create teams that cut across from outpatient services to inpatient and residential services. We realized that when a youngster was receiving outpatient treatment and had a crisis that required a more structured and controlled environment, we often hit a crossroad in treatment. Too often the family would become hopeless because of the new crisis and consider leaving treatment. We must admit that this same sentiment was also experienced by our therapists who were feeling helpless in preventing the crisis. Just as family members of adolescents may experience hopelessness, so can therapists become discouraged by uneven progress and unexpected relapses and hospitalizations. The transition in our way of thinking that was needed was to see these setbacks as a natural part of the therapy process. We worked to remove the hopelessness from the situation (on both the family and treatment team side) and to figure out ways to ensure that the teams continue to work together. In this way we avoid the perception that treatment has failed, that the family must start anew with another treatment team, or that it is best to give up on the therapy and the youth completely. By reframing the situation away from another failure to a consistent therapeutic situation that integrates the crisis points, the family and adolescent can continue to be supported and continue to grow. When we were able to establish a strong relationship between our family treatment team and the residential or crisis teams, there was seamless support across the systems and the youth and families benefited. When the youth was hospitalized or in short-term residential, the family could often benefit from continued family services that instilled hope and prepared them for the youth's re-entry into the family. Our therapists were also often allowed to come onto the units to continue to teach the crisis management, emotion regulation, and distress tolerance skills based on DBT work (Fruzzetti et al., 2021; Linehan 1993, 2014a, 2014b, in press-a, in press-b) or to conduct family sessions. This solidified the idea that this was all part of one larger therapeutic process.

CONCLUSION AND FUTURE DIRECTIONS

Our Culturally Informed and Flexible Family-Based Treatment for Adolescents (CIFFTA) creates a foundation with a strong systemic and contextual perspective, which is informed by cultural uniqueness, and that flexes to clearly identify the unique circumstances that will inform the tailoring of treatment to the family. In this chapter, we shared experiences that led to extensions of CIFFTA's work and a widening of the treatment lens so that we could meet the needs of new populations.

Although not as extensive as the work we have done with Latine populations, our work with African American, Haitian, and other Black populations has continued and is enriching our approach. This work requires a willingness and ability to call out the structural and systemic inequities that exist and ensure that our work does not collude with these systems. It means helping family members to mobilize their protective processes to support each other as they face these chronic multigenerational stressors. In this work we must take a strength-based approach and fight the tendency to be overly pathology-focused. It is important that the therapy provide tools for addressing minority stressors such as racism, discrimination, and anti-immigrant messages that undermine the well-being of all family members. By doing this, the treatment becomes increasingly ecologically valid (Bernal & Scharron-del Rio, 2001). Although it is easy for the therapist to conceptually be prepared for these difficult issues, it is important that they be prepared, confident, and comfortable with the delivery of the information in sessions. This is a separate and important step that can be facilitated by having written content as part of the treatment manual and ensuring that therapists *practice* communicating these important messages in their own words. We hope that we have shown how this work is integrated and not separate from the individual and family mechanisms of action (e.g., the enhancement of motivation, skills, and family functioning).

We are enthusiastic about future developments that we have planned for CIFFTA and that will support the work of the dedicated counselors and therapists who can make a difference in our community. Just as we shared our use of technology as a disruptive force to rethink our ways of training and coaching, we hope to integrate technology into the tools we provide therapists. A very promising approach is to create engaging and therapy-enhancing videos that can create readiness to learn and use the psychoeducational modules (Santisteban et al., 2017). This is based on the idea that easy to use and engaging tools can give the therapist more options for delivering helpful material. Our CIFFTA team is dedicated to continued growth in response to client, therapist, and organization's workforce needs.

We began this book by stating that a strength of family therapy is that it uses a contextual and relational approach that looks at the relationship dynamics that influence individual and family behaviors. Throughout this book the relational approach has guided us to reflect on the complex contexts (e.g., schools, neighborhoods, health systems, immigration policies) that directly impact the well-being of both adolescents and families. At the same time as we look at larger structural and systemic issues, we also look within the family for culture-related processes that impact well-being and the treatment process. The integration of cultural values and worldviews has been a hallmark of family therapy (Boyd-Franklin, 2010; Falicov, 2014; McGoldrick & Hardy, 2019) even though this strength has not always been reflected in the more formal evidence-based treatments that emphasize only treatment mechanisms while avoiding the interaction of culture and mechanisms (Santisteban et al., 2013). This narrow view may fail to address the unique life experiences that contribute to hopelessness, stressors, and poor service utilization that we are charged with changing (Abraído-Lanza et al., 2016). Throughout this book we have argued that these experiences are a starting point in therapy so that culture-related experiences and mechanisms of change are two threads running through the same discussion and therapeutic work. We started this book with the goal of showing the reader how our mechanisms of action at the individual and family levels can be integrated with a cultural, relational, and contextual perspective that is constantly accounting for the unique life experiences of minoritized populations. We hope that we have met this goal at least in part and that we have whet your appetite to continue to learn, develop, and grow in the truly meaningful work you do.

References

Aarons, G. A., Wells, R. S., Zagursky, K., Fettes, D. L., & Palinkas, L. A. (2009). Implementing evidence-based practice in community mental health agencies: A multiple stakeholder analysis. *American Journal of Public Health, 99*(11), 2087–2095.

Abraído-Lanza, A. F, Echeverría, S. E., & Flórez, K. R. (2016). Latino immigrants, acculturation, and health: Promising new directions in research. *Annual Review of Public Health, 37*(1), 219–236.

Abrams, M. S. (2015). Coming together to move apart: Family therapy for enhancing adolescent development. *American Journal of Psychotherapy, 69*(3), 285–299.

Alegría, M., Alvarez, K., Ishikawa, R. Z., DiMarzio, K., & McPeck, S. (2016). Removing obstacles to eliminating racial and ethnic disparities in behavioral health care. *Health Affairs (Project Hope), 35*(6), 991–999.

Amaro, H., Raj, A., Reed, E., & Cranston, K. (2002). Implementation and long-term outcomes of two HIV intervention programs for Latinas. *Health Promotion Practice, 3*(2), 245–254.

American Psychiatric Association (APA). (2000). *Diagnostic and statistical manual of mental disorders* (4th ed., text rev.). Author.

American Psychiatric Association (APA). (2013). Cultural formulation. In American Psychiatric Association, *Diagnostic and statistical manual of mental disorders* (5th ed., text rev., pp. 860–871). Author.

Aneshensel, C. S. (1992). Social stress: Theory and research. *Annual Review of Sociology, 18,* 15–38.

Backer, T. E. (2000). The failure of success: Challenges of disseminating effective substance abuse prevention programs. *Journal of Community Psychology, 28*(3), 363–373.

Bagley, S. M., Anderson, B. J., & Stein, M. D. (2017). Usefulness of the CRAFFT to diagnose alcohol or cannabis use disorders in a sample of emerging adults with past-month alcohol or cannabis use. *Journal of Child and Adolescent Substance Abuse, 26* (1), 18–23.

Baker, B. L., Heller, T. L., & Blacher, J. (1995). Staff attitudes toward family involvement in residential treatment centers for children. *Psychiatric Services, 46,* 60–65.

Beidas, R. S., & Kendall, P. C. (2010). Training therapists in evidence-based practice: A critical review of studies from a systems-contextual perspective. *Clinical Psychology: Science and Practice, 17*(1), 1–30.

Berger Cardoso, J., Goldbach, J. T., Cervantes, R. C., & Swank, P. (2016). Stress and multiple substance use behaviors among Hispanic adolescents. *Prevention Science, 17*(2), 208–217.

Bergmann, J., Overmyer, J., & Wilie, B. (2012, April 14). *The flipped class: Myths vs. reality.* The Daily Riff. Retrieved from https://kmtrosclair.wordpress.com/wp-content/uploads/2015/06/the-flipped-class-myths-vs-reality-the-daily-riff-be-smarter-about-education.pdf

Bermudez, J. M., & Mancini, J. (2013). "Familias Fuertes": Resilience among Latino families. In D. Becvar (Ed.), *Handbook of family resilience* (pp. 215–227). Springer.

Bernal, G., & Domenech Rodríguez, M. M. (2012). *Cultural adaptations: Tools for evidence-based practice with diverse populations.* American Psychological Association.

Bernal, G., & Scharron-Del-Rio, M. R. (2001). Are empirically supported treatments valid for ethnic minorities? Toward an alternative approach for treatment research. *Cultural Diversity and Ethnic Minority Psychology, 7,* 328–342.

Berry, J. W. (1991). Understanding and managing multiculturalism. *Journal of Psychology and Developing Societies, 3,* 17–49.

Berry, J. W. (1992). Cultural transformation and psychological acculturation. In J. Burnet, D. Juteau, E. Padolsky, A. Rasporich, & A. Sirois (Eds.), *Migration and the transformation of cultures* (pp. 23–54). Multicultural History Society of Ontario.

Berry, J. W. (2005). Acculturation: Living successfully in two cultures. *International Journal of Intercultural Relations, 29*(6), 697–712.

Berry, J. W. (2006). Contexts of acculturation. In D. L. Sam & J. W. Berry (Eds.), *Cambridge handbook of acculturation psychology* (pp. 27–42). Cambridge University Press.

Berry, J. W., & Sam, D. (1996). Acculturation and adaptation. In J. W. Berry, M. H. Segall, & C. Kagitcibasi (Eds.), *Handbook of cross-cultural psychology: Vol. 3. Social behavior and applications.* Allyn & Bacon.

Bischoff, R. J., Hollist, C. S., Smith, C. W., & Flack, P. (2004). Addressing the mental health needs of the rural underserved: Findings from a multiple case study of a behavioral telehealth Project. *Contemporary Family Therapy: An International Journal, 26,* 179–198.

Bitter, J. R. (2014). *Theory and practice of family therapy and counseling* (2nd ed.). Brooks/Cole Cengage Learning.

Blasé, K. A. (2007, February). *Factors that contribute to successful implementation.* Presentation at the American Family Therapy Academy, Clinical Research Conference, Miami Lakes, FL.

Bostwick, W. B., Meyer, I., Aranda, F., Russell, S., Hughes, T., Birkett, M., & Mustanski, B. (2014). Mental health and suicidality among racially/ethnically diverse sexual minority youths. *American Journal of Public Health, 104*, 1129–1136.

Boyd-Franklin, N. (2003). *Black families in therapy: Understanding the African American experience* (2nd ed.). Guilford Press.

Boyd-Franklin, N. (2010). Incorporating spirituality and religion into the treatment of African American clients. *Counseling Psychologist, 38*(7), 976–1000.

Brietzke, M., & Perreira, K. (2017). Stress and coping: Latino youth coming of age in a new Latino destination. *Journal of Adolescent Research, 32*(4), 407–432.

Bronfenbrenner, U. (2005). *Making human beings human: Bioecological perspectives on human development.* SAGE.

Burton, M., & Guzzo, R. (2020). Liberation psychology: Origins and development. In L. Comas-Díaz & E. Torres Rivera (Eds.), *Liberation psychology: Theory, method, practice, and social justice* (pp. 17–40). American Psychological Association.

Caetano, R., Ramisetty-Mikler, S., Caetano Vaeth, P. A., & Harris, T. R. (2007). Acculturation stress, drinking, and intimate partner violence among Hispanic couples in the U.S. *Journal of Interpersonal Violence, 22*(11), 1431–1447.

Calderón-Tena, C. O., Knight, G. P., & Carlo, G. (2011). The socialization of prosocial behavioral tendencies among Mexican American adolescents: The role of familism values. *Cultural Diversity and Ethnic Minority Psychology, 17*(1), 98–106.

Carter, E. A., & McGoldrick, M. (1999). *The expanded family life cycle: Individual, family, and social perspectives* (3rd ed.). Allyn & Bacon.

Casares, M. Á., Díez-Gómez, A., Pérez-Albéniz, A., Lucas-Molina, B., & Fonseca-Pedrero, E. (2024). Screening for anxiety in adolescents: Validation of the Generalized Anxiety Disorder Assessment –7 in a representative sample of adolescents. *Journal of Affective Disorders, 354*, 331–338.

Castro, F. G., & Alarcón, E. H. (2002). Integrating cultural variables into drug abuse prevention and treatment with racial/ethnic minorities. *Journal of Drug Issues, 32*, 783–810.

Castro, F. G., Barrera, J. M., & Martinez, J. C. R. (2004). The cultural adaptation of prevention interventions: Resolving tensions between fidelity and fit. *Prevention Science, 5*(1), 41–45.

Castro, F. G., Stein, J. A., & Bentler, P. M. (2009). Ethnic pride, traditional family values and acculturation in early cigarette and alcohol use among Latino adolescents. *Journal of Primary Prevention, 30*, 265–292.

Cela, T., Marcelin, H., Waldman, R., Dembo, R., Demezier, D., Clement, R., . . . Hogue, A. (2023). Haitian and Haitian American experiences of racism and socioethnic discrimination in Miami-Dade county: At-risk and court-involved youth. *Family Process, 62*(1), 216–229.

Centers for Disease Control and Prevention. (2016). *Reduced disparities in* birth rates among teens aged 15–19 years—United States, 2006–2007 and 2013–2014. Retrieved from *www.cdc.gov/mmwr/volumes/65/wr/mm6516a1.htm*

Cervantes, R. C. (2017). *A guide for conducting clinical assessment of Hispanic and Latino clients.* SAMHSA Center for Substance Abuse Treatment, National Hispanic and Latino Addiction Technology Transfer Center.

Cervantes, R. C., Berger Cardoso, J., & Goldbach, J. T. (2015). Examining differences in culturally based stress among clinical and non-clinical Hispanic adolescents. *Cultural Diversity and Ethnic Minority Psychology, 21*(3), 458–467.

Cervantes, R. C., & Bui, T. (2015). Culturally informed psychosocial stress assessment for Hispanics. In K. F. Geisinger (Ed.), *Psychological testing of Hispanics: Clinical, cultural, and intellectual issues* (2nd ed., pp. 273–289). American Psychological Association.

Cervantes, R. C., Fisher, D. G., Córdova, D., & Napper, L. E. (2011). The Hispanic Stress Inventory—Adolescent Version: A culturally informed psychosocial assessment. *Psychological Assessment. Psychological Assessment, 24*(1), 187–196.

Cervantes, R. C., Fisher, D. G., Padilla, A. M., & Napper, L. E. (2016). The Hispanic Stress Inventory–Version 2: Improving the assessment of acculturation stress. *Psychological Assessment, 28*(5), 509–522.

Cervantes, R. C., Gattamorta, K. A., & Berger-Cardoso, J. (2018). Examining difference in immigration stress, acculturation stress and mental health outcomes in six Hispanic/Latino nativity and regional groups. *Journal of Immigrant and Minority Health, 21*(1), 14–20.

Cervantes, R. C., Goldbach, J., & Padilla, A. (2012). Using qualitative methods for revising the Hispanic Stress Inventory. *Hispanic Journal of Behavioral Sciences, 34*(2), 208–231.

Cervantes, R. C., Goldbach, J. T., Varela, A., & Santisteban, D. A. (2014). Self-harm among Hispanic adolescents: Investigating the role of culture-related stressors. *Journal of Adolescent Health, 55*(5), 633–639.

Cervantes, R. C., Gonzalez-Guarda, R. M., McCabe, B. E., & Nagy, G. A. (2023). Measuring Hispanic optimism and personal expectancy. *Hispanic Journal of Behavioral Sciences, 44*(4), 267–296.

Cervantes, R. C., Padilla, A., & Salgado de Snyder, N. (1991). The Hispanic Stress Inventory: A culturally relevant approach to psychosocial assessment. *Journal of Consulting and Clinical Psychology, 3*(3), 438–447.

Cervantes, R. C., & Santisteban, D. S. (2016, June 1–3). *Enhancing family resilience among at risk Latinos.* Panel Presentation, Presented at the Society for Prevention Research Annual Conference, San Francisco, CA.

Christensen, L. L. (1995). Therapists' perspectives on home-based family therapy. *American Journal of Family Therapy, 23*(4), 301–314.

Clermont-Mathieu, M., & Nicholas, G. (2016). Parenting practices and culture in Haiti. In G. Nicholas, A. Bejaramo, & D. L. Lee (Eds.), *Contemporary parenting: A global perspective* (pp. 95–104). Routledge.

Coatsworth, J. D., Santisteban, D. A., McBride, C. K., & Szapocznik, J. (2001). Brief strategic family therapy versus community control: Engagement, retention, and an exploration of the moderating role of adolescent symptom severity. *Family Process, 40*(3), 313–332.

Coleman, B. W., Horsford, S., Norton, E. H., Adams, A., Lee, S. J., Omar, I., . . . Lewis, J. (2019). *Ring the alarm: The crisis of Black youth suicide in America.* A report to Congress from the Congressional Black Caucus, Washington, DC.

Constantino, M. J., Coyne, A. E., Boswell, J. F., Iles, B. R., & Visla, A. (2018). A meta-analysis of the association between patients' early perception of treatment credibility and their posttreatment outcomes. *Psychotherapy, 55,* 486–495.

Convertino, A. D., Helm, J. L., Pennesi, J. L., Gonzales, M., 4th, & Blashill, A. J. (2021). Integrating minority stress theory and the tripartite influence model: A model of eating disordered behavior in sexual minority young adults. *Appetite, 163,* 105204.

Cortés, D. E., Rogler, L. H., & Malgady, R. G. (1994). Biculturality among Puerto Rican adults in the United States. *American Journal of Community Psychology, 5,* 707–721.

Cox, R. B., Burr, B., Blow, A. J., & Parra Cardona, J. R. (2011). Latino adolescent substance use in the United States: Using the bioecodevelopmental model as an organizing framework for research and practice. *Journal of Family Theory and Review, 3*(2), 96–123.

Cyrus, K. (2017). Multiple minorities as multiply marginalized: Applying the minority stress theory to LGBTQ people of color. *Journal of Gay and Lesbian Mental Health, 21*(3), 194–202.

Dansereau, D. F., & Dees, S. M. (2002). Mapping training: The transfer of a cognitive technology for improving counseling. *Journal of Substance Abuse Treatment, 22,* 219–230.

Detjen, G. M., Nieto, J. F., Trentthiem-Dietz, A., Fleming, M., & Chasan-Taber, L. (2007). Acculturation and cigarette smoking among pregnant Hispanic women residing in the United States. *American Journal of Public Health, 97*(11), 2040–2047.

Doherty, W. J. (1995). Boundaries between parent and family education and family therapy: The levels of family involvement model. *Family relations, 44*(4), 353–358.

Dohrenwend, B. P. (2000). The role of adversity and stress in psychopathology: Some evidence and its implications for theory and research. *Journal of Health and Social Behavior, 41*(1), 1–19.

Donato, K. M. (2010). US migration from Latin America: Gendered patterns and shifts. *Annals of the American Academy of Political and Social Science, 630*(1), 78–92.

Donovan, J. E., & Jessor, R. (1985). Structure of problem behavior in adolescence and young adulthood. *Journal of consulting and clinical Psychology, 53*(6), 890–904.

Evans, A., & Kaiser, S. (2022). *When faith meets therapy: Finding hope and a practical path to emotional, spiritual, and relational healing.* Thomas Nelson.

Evans, G. W., & Kim, P. (2007). Childhood poverty and health: Cumulative risk exposure and stress dysregulation. *Psychological Science, 18,* 953–957.

Falicov, C. J. (2014). *Latino families in therapy* (2nd ed.). Guilford Press.

Falicov, C. J. (2017). Multidimensional ecosystemic comparative approach (MECA). In J. L. Lebow, A. Chambers, & D. C. Breunlin (Eds.), *Encyclopedia of couple and family therapy.* Springer.

Fishman, H. (2022). *Performance-based family therapy: A therapist's guide to measurable change.* Routledge.

Fixsen, D. L., Naoom, S. F., Blasé, K. A., Friedman, R. M., & Wallace, F. (2005). *Implementation research: A synthesis of the literature* (Publication No. 231). Louis de la Parte Florida Mental Health Institute.

Foxen, P. (2016). *Mental health services for Latino youth: Bridging culture and evidence.* National Council of La Raza.

Fraenkel, P. (2023). *Last chance couple therapy: Bringing relationships back from the brink.* Norton.

Fruzzetti, A. E., Payne, L. G., & Hoffman, P. D. (2021). DBT with families. In L. A. Dimeff & K. Koerner (Eds.), *Dialectical behavior therapy in clinical practice: Applications across disorders and settings* (2nd ed., pp. 366–387). Guilford Press.

Fry, R., & Passel, J. S. (2009). *Latino children: A majority are U.S.-born offspring of immigrants.* Pew Hispanic Center.

Gallo, L. C., Penedo, F. J., De los Monteros, K., & Arguelles, W. (2009). Resiliency in the face of disadvantage: Do Hispanic cultural characteristics protect health outcomes? *Journal of Personality, 77*(6), 1707–1746.

Gamble, V. (1993). A legacy of distrust: African Americans and medical research. *American Journal of Preventive Medicine, 9,* 35–38.

Geisinger, K. (Ed.). (2015). *Psychological testing of Hispanics: Clinical and intellectual issues.* American Psychological Association Press.

Germán, M., Gonzales, N. A., & Dumka, L. (2009). Familism values as a protective factor for Mexican-origin adolescents exposed to deviant peers. *Journal of Early Adolescence, 29*(1), 16–42.

Glebova, T., Foster, S. L., Cunningham, P. B., Brennan, P. A., & Whitmore, E. (2012). Examining therapist comfort in delivering family therapy in home and community settings: Development and evaluation of the Therapist Comfort Scale. *Psychotherapy, 49*(1), 52–61.

Goldbach, J. T., Berger Cardoso, J., Cervantes, R. C., & Duan, L. (2015). The relation between stress and alcohol use among Hispanic adolescents. *Psychology of Addictive Behaviors, 29*(4), 960–968.

Goldbach, J. T., & Gibbs, J. (2015). Strategies employed by sexual minority adolescents to cope with minority stress. *Psychology of Sexual Orientation and Gender Diversity, 2,* 297–306.

Goldbach, J. T., Tanner-Smith, E. E., Bagwell, M., & Dunlap, S. (2014). Minority stress and substance use in sexual minority adolescents: A meta-analysis. *Prevention Science, 15*(3), 350–363.

Gulbas, L. E., Guz, S., Hausmann-Stabile, C., Szlyk, H. S., & Zayas, L. H. (2019). Trajectories of well-being among Latin adolescents who attempt suicide: A longitudinal qualitative analysis. *Qualitative Health Research, 29*(12), 1766–1780.

Hailey, J., Burton, W., & Arscott, J. (2020). We are family: Chosen and created families as a protective factor against racialized trauma and anti-LGBTQ oppression among African American sexual and gender minority youth. *Journal of GLBT Family Studies, 16*(2), 176–191.

Hall, G. C., N., Ibaraki, A. Y., Huang, E. R., Marti, C. N., & Stice, E. (2016). A meta-analysis of cultural adaptations of psychological interventions. *Behavior Therapy, 47*(6), 993–1014.

Harrell, S. P. (2000). A multidimensional conceptualization of racism-related stress: Implications for the well-being of people of color. *American Journal of Orthopsychiatry, 70*(1), 42–57.

Harrison, K. L. (2021). A call to action: Online learning and distance education in the training of couple and family therapists. *Journal of Marital and Family Therapy, 47*(2), 408–423.

Ho, M. K., Rasheed, J. M., & Rasheed, M. N. (2004). *Family therapy with ethnic minorities* (2nd ed.). SAGE.

Hofstede, G. (1980). *Culture's consequences: International differences in work related values.* SAGE.

Hogue, A., Becker, S. J., Wenzel, K., Henderson, C. E., Bobek, M., Levy, S., & Fishman, M. (2021). Family involvement in treatment and recovery for substance use disorders among transition-age youth: Research bedrocks and opportunities. *Journal of Substance Abuse Treatment, 129,* 108402.

Horvath, A. O., & Greenberg, L. S. (1994). *The working alliance: Theory, research, and practice.* Wiley.

Hughes, L. (1994). *The collected poems of Langston Hughes.* Knopf.

Human Rights Campaign & League of United Latin American Citizens. (2012). *Supporting and caring for our Latino LGBT youth.* Author.

Institute of Medicine. (2007). *The state of quality improvement and implementation research: Workshop summary.* National Academies Press.

Institute of Medicine Committee on Community-Based Drug Treatment. (1998). *Bridging the gap between practice and research: Forging partnerships with community-based drug and alcohol treatment* (S. Lamb, M. R. Greenlick, & D. McCarty, Eds.). National Academies Press.

Institute of Medicine & National Research Council. (2014). *The National Children's Study 2014: An assessment.* National Academies Press.

Ivey-Stephenson, A. Z., Demissie, Z., Crosby, A. E., Stone, D. M., Gaylor, E., Wilkins, N., . . . Brown, M. (2020). Suicidal ideation and behaviors among high school students—Youth Risk Behavior Survey, United States, 2019. *Morbidity and Mortality Weekly Report, 69*(Suppl. 1), 47–55.

Jackson, C. B., Quetsch, L. B., Brabson, L. A., & Herschell, A. D. (2018). Web-based training methods for behavioral health providers: A systematic review. *Administration and Policy in Mental Health and Mental Health Services Research, 45.* 587–610.

Jessor, R., & Jessor, S. L. (1977). *Problem behavior and psychosocial development: A longitudinal study of youth.* Academic Press.

Joe, S., Romer, D., & Jamieson, P. E. (2007). Suicide acceptability is related to suicide planning in U.S. adolescents and young adults. *Suicide and Life-Threatening Behavior, 37*(2), 165–178.

Jones, S. C. T., & Neblett, E. W. (2017). Future directions in research on racism-related stress and racial-ethnic protective factors for Black youth. *Journal of Clinical Child and Adolescent Psychology, 46*(5), 754–766.

Jurist, E. (2018). *Minding emotions: Cultivating mentalization in psychotherapy.* Guilford Press.

Kann, L., McManus, T., Harris, W. A., Shanklin, S. L., Flint, K. H., Queen, B., . . . Ethier, K. A. (2018). Youth Risk Behavior Surveillance—United States, 2017. *Morbidity and Mortality Weekly Reports Surveillance Summary, 67*(SS-8), 1–114.

Kaslow, N. J., Broth, M. R., Smith, C. O., & Collins, M. H. (2012). Family-based interventions for child and adolescent disorders. *Journal of Marital and Family Therapy, 38*(1), 82–100.

Kendall, P. C., Gosch, E., Furr, J. M., & Sood, E. (2008). Flexibility with fidelity. *Journal of the American Academy of Child and Adolescent Psychiatry, 47,* 987–993.

Kluckhohn, F. R., & Strodtbeck, F. L. (1961). *Variations in value orientations.* Row, Peterson.

Koss-Chioino, J., & Vargas, L. A. (1999). *Working with Latino youth: Culture, development, and context* (1st ed.). Jossey-Bass.

Laszloffy, T. A., & Hardy, K. V. (2000). Uncommon strategies for a common problem: Addressing racism in family therapy. *Family Process, 39*(1), 35–50.

Lazarus, R. S., & Folkman, S. (1984). *Stress, appraisal, and coping.* Springer.

Linehan, M. M. (1993). *Cognitive-behavioral treatment of borderline personality disorder.* Guilford Press.

Linehan, M. M. (2014a). *DBT skills training handouts and worksheets* (2nd ed.). Guilford Press.

Linehan, M. M. (2014b). *DBT skills training manual* (2nd ed.). Guilford Press.

Linehan, M. M. (in press-a). *DBT skills training handouts and worksheets* (rev. ed.). Guilford Press.

Linehan, M. M. (in press-b). *DBT skills training manual* (rev. ed.). Guilford Press.

Marcelin, L. H. (2012). In the name of the nation: Ritual, blood, and the political habitus of violence in Haiti. *American Anthropologist, 114*(2), 253–266.

Marín, G., & Marín, B. V. (1991). *Research with Hispanic populations.* SAGE.

Markiewicz, J., Ebert, L., Ling, D., Amaya-Jackson, L., & Kisiel, C. (2006). *Learning collaborative toolkit.* National Center for Child Traumatic Stress.

Marks, A. K., Kida, E., & García Coll, C. (2014). Understanding the

U.S. immigrant paradox in childhood and adolescence. *Child Development Perspectives, 8*(2), 59–64.

Marsiglia, F. F., Parsai, M. B., & Kulis, S. (2009). Effects of familism & family cohesion on problem behaviors among adolescents in Mexican immigrant families in the southwest U.S. *Journal of Ethnicity and Cultural Diversity in Social Work, 18,* 203–220.

Mason, C. A., Cauce, A. M., Gonzales, N., & Hiraga, Y. (1996). Neither too sweet nor too sour: Problem peers, maternal control, and problem behavior in African American adolescents. *Child Development, 67*(5), 2115–2130.

Masten, A. S., & Cicchetti, D. (2016). Resilience in development: Progress and transformation. In D. Cicchetti (Ed.), *Developmental psychopathology: Risk, resilience, and intervention* (3rd ed., pp. 271–333). Wiley.

McGoldrick, M., Gerson, R., & Shellenberger, S. (1999). *Genograms: assessment and intervention* (2nd ed.). Norton.

McGoldrick, M., & Hardy, K. V. (2019). *Re-visioning family therapy: Addressing diversity in clinical practice* (3rd ed.). Guilford Press.

McHugh, R. K., & Barlow, D. H. (2010). The dissemination and implementation of evidence-based psychological interventions: A review of current efforts. *American Psychologist, 73,* 73–84.

McHugh, R. K., Murray, H. W., & Barlow, D. H. (2009). Balancing fidelity and adaptation in the dissemination of empirically-supported treatments: The promise of transdiagnostic interventions. *Behaviour Research and Therapy, 47*(11), 946–953.

Mena, M. P., del Rey, G. M., Gutierrez, M., Gattamorta, K., Lazarus, R. A., & Santisteban, D. A. (2024a). *Culturally informed and flexible family based treatment for adolescents: Integrating technology and modular content that facilitates treatment tailoring to better serve adolescents with self-harm behavior.* Unpublished manuscript.

Mena, M. P., Dillon, F. R., Mason, C. A., & Santisteban, D. A. (2008a). Communication about sexually related topics among Hispanic substance-abusing adolescents and their parents. *Journal of Drug Issues, 38*(1), 215–234.

Mena, M. P., Lazarus, R. A., Otero, K. A., & Santisteban, D. A. (2024b). Evaluation of culturally informed and flexible family-based treatment for adolescents (CIFFTA) implemented in community-based settings. *Journal of Community Psychology, 52*(2), 363–381.

Mena, M. P., Mason, C., Santisteban, D. A. (2023). *Extended parent–child separations: Impact on adolescent functioning and possible gender differences.* Unpublished Manuscript.

Mena, M. P., Mitrani, V. B., Muir, J. A., & Santisteban, D. A. (2008b). Extended parent-child separations: Impact on substance-abusing Hispanic adolescents. *Journal for Specialists in Pediatric Nursing, 13*(1), 50–52.

Meyer, I. H. (2003). Prejudice, social stress, and mental health in lesbian, gay, and bisexual populations: Conceptual issues and research evidence. *Psychological Bulletin, 129*(5), 674–697.

Miller, W. R., & Rollnick, S. (2023). *Motivational interviewing: Helping people change and grow* (4th ed.). Guilford Press.

Minuchin, S., & Fishman, H. C. (1981). *Family therapy techniques*. Harvard University Press.

Mitrani, V. B., Santisteban, D. A., & Muir, J. A. (2004). Addressing immigration-related separations in Hispanic families with a behavior-problem adolescent. *American Journal of Orthopsychiatry, 74*(3), 219–229.

Moffitt, T. E., & Caspi, A. (2001). Childhood predictors differentiate life-course persistent and adolescence-limited antisocial pathways among males and females. *Development and Psychopathology, 13*(2), 355–375.

Morcillo, C., Duarte, C. S., Shen, S., Blanco, C., Canino, G., & Bird, H. R. (2011). Parental familism and antisocial behaviors: Development, gender, and potential mechanisms. *Journal of the American Academy of Child and Adolescent Psychiatry, 50*, 471–479.

Mueller, A. S., James, W., Abrutyn, S., & Levin, M. L. (2015). Suicide ideation and bullying among US adolescents: Examining the intersections of sexual orientation, gender, and race/ethnicity. *American Journal of Public Health, 105*, 980–985.

Murray, B. A. (2014). The use of high-fidelity simulation in psychiatric and mental health nursing clinical education. *International Journal of Health Sciences Education, 2*(1).

Naar-King, S. (2011). Motivational interviewing in adolescent treatment. *Canadian Journal of Psychiatry, 56*(11), 651–657.

Nadeem, E., Gleacher, A., & Beidas, R. S. (2013). Consultation as an implementation strategy for evidence-based practices across multiple contexts: Unpacking the black box. *Administration and Policy in Mental Health and Mental Health Services Research, 40*(6), 439–450.

National Academies of Sciences, Engineering, and Medicine. (2019a). *The promise of adolescence: Realizing opportunity for all youth*. National Academies Press.

National Academies of Sciences, Engineering, and Medicine. (2019b). *Fostering healthy mental, emotional, and behavioral development in children and youth: A national agenda*. National Academies Press.

Nelson, T. S., Chenail, R. J., Alexander, J. F., Crane, D. R., Johnson, S. M., & Schwallie, L. (2007). The development of core competencies for the practice of marriage and family therapy. *Journal of Marital and Family Therapy, 33*(4), 417–438.

Noé-Bustamante, L., Mora, L., & Lopez, M. H. (2020, August 11). *About one-in-four U.S. Hispanics have heard of Latinx, but just 3% use it*. Pew Research Center. Retrieved from www.pewresearch.org/race-and-ethnicity/2020/08/11/about-one-in-four-u-s-hispanics-have-heard-of-latinx-but-just-3-use-it

Novins, D. K., Green, A. E., Legha, R. K., & Aarons, G. A. (2013). Dissemination and implementation of evidence-based practices for child and adolescent mental health: A systematic review. *Journal of the American Academy of Child and Adolescent Psychiatry, 52*(10), 1009–1025.

Oesterle, T. S., Hitschfeld, M. J., Lineberry, T. W., & Schneekloth, T. D. (2015). CRAFFT as a substance use screening instrument for adolescent psychiatry admissions. *Journal of Psychiatric Practice, 21*(4), 259–266.

Oliver, J. A., & Lang, J. M. (2018). Barriers and consultation needs regarding implementation of evidence-based treatment in community agencies. *Children and Youth Services Review, 94*, 368–377.

Palmer, R. H. C., Young, S. E., Hopfer, C. J., Corley, R. P., Stallings, M. C., Crowley, T. J., & Hewitt, J. K. (2009). Developmental epidemiology of drug use and abuse in adolescence and young adulthood: Evidence of generalized risk. *Drug and Alcohol Dependence, 102*(1), 78–87.

Patterson, G. R. (1982). *Coercive family process*. Castalia.

Powell, B. J., McMillen, J. C., Hawley, K. M., & Proctor, E. K. (2013). Mental health clinicians' motivation to invest in training: Results from a practice-based research network survey. *Psychiatric Services, 64*(8), 816–818.

Price, J. H., & Khubchandani, J. (2019). The changing characteristics of African American adolescent suicides, 2001–2017. *Journal of Community Health, 44*, 756–763.

Prochaska, J. O., & DiClemente, C. C. (1992). Stages of change in the modification of problem behaviors. In M. Hersen, R. M. Eisler, & P. M. Miller (Eds.), *Progress in behavior modification* (pp. 184–214). Sycamore Press.

Radillo, R. M. (2007). *Cuidado pastoral: Contextual e integral*. Libros Desafío.

Randell, N. G. (2012). Practice, practice, practice: Preliminary findings from an evidence-based practice funding initiative at the Peter and Elizabeth C. Tower Foundation. *Foundation Review, 4*(2), 14–29.

Rastogi, M., Massey-Hastings, N., & Wieling, E. (2012). Barriers to seeking mental health services in the Latino/a community: A qualitative analysis. *Journal of Systemic Therapies, 31*(4), 1–17.

Richardson, L. P., McCauley, E., Grossman, D. C., McCarty, C. A., Richards, J., Russo, J. E., Rockhill, C., & Katon, W. (2010). Evaluation of the Patient Health Questionnaire–9 Item for detecting major depression among adolescents. *Pediatrics, 126*(6), 1117–1123.

Ríos-Ellis, B., Aguilar-Gaxiola, S., Cabassa, L., Caetano, R., Comas-Díaz, L., Flores, Y., . . . Ugarte, C. (2005). *Critical disparities in Latino mental health: Transforming research into action* (White Paper). Institute for Hispanic Health, NCLR (National Council of La Raza).

Robbins, M. S, Alexander, J. F, Newell, R. M, & Turner, C. W. (1996). The immediate effect of reframing on client attitude in family therapy. *Journal of Family Psychology, 10*(1), 28–34.

Robinson, S. M., Sobell, L. C., Sobell, M. B., & Leo, G. I. (2014). Reliability of the Timeline Followback for cocaine, cannabis, and cigarette use. *Psychology of Addictive Behaviors, 28* (1), 154–162.

Roh, K. H., & Park, H. (2010). A meta-analysis on the effectiveness of computer-based education in nursing. *Healthcare Informatics Research, 16*(3), 149–157.

Romero, A. J., & Roberts, R. E. (2003). Stress within a bicultural context for adolescents of Mexican descent. *Cultural Diversity and Ethnic Minority Psychology, 9,* 171–184.

Rosa, E. M., & Tudge, J. (2013). Urie Bronfenbrenner's theory of human development: Its evolution from ecology to bioecology. *Journal of Family Theory and Review, 5*(4), 243–258.

Rosenthal, L. (2016). Incorporating intersectionality into psychology: An opportunity to promote social justice and equity. *American Psychologist, 71*(6), 474–485.

Rudmin, F. W. (2009). Constructs, measurements and models of acculturation and acculturative stress. *International Journal of Intercultural Relations, 33,* 106–123.

Rumbaut, R. G. (2008). Reaping what you sow: Immigration, youth, and reactive ethnicity. *Applied Developmental Science, 12*(2), 108–111.

Ryan, C. (2010). Engaging families to support lesbian, gay, bisexual and transgender (LGBT) youth: The Family Acceptance Project. *Prevention Researcher, 17*(4), 11–13.

Sabogal, F., Marin, G., Otero-Sabogal, R., & Marin, B. (1987). Hispanic familism and acculturation: What changes and what doesn't? *Hispanic Journal of Behavioral Sciences, 9*(4), 397–412.

Sam, D. L., & Berry, J. W. (2010). Acculturation: When individuals and groups of different cultural backgrounds meet. *Perspectives on Psychological Science, 5,* 472–481.

Santa-Maria, M. L., & Cornille, T. (2007). Traumatic stress, family separations, and attachment among Latin American immigrants. *Traumatology (Tallahassee, Fla.), 13*(2), 26–31.

Santisteban, D. A. (2008). *Engaging reluctant family members into adolescent's substance abuse treatment: A guide for practitioners.* Southern Coast Addiction Technology Transfer Center.

Santisteban, D. A., Coatsworth, J. D., Perez-Vidal, A., Kurtines, W. M., Schwartz, S. J., LaPerriere, A., & Szapocznik, J. (2003). Efficacy of brief strategic family therapy in modifying Hispanic adolescent behavior problems and substance use. *Journal of Family Psychology, 17*(1), 121–133.

Santisteban, D. A., Czaja, S. J., Nair, S. N., Mena, M. P., & Tulloch, A. R. (2017). Computer assisted culturally informed flexible family based treatment for adolescents: A randomized clinical trial for at-risk racial/ethnic minority adolescents. *Behavior Therapy, 48*(4), 474–489.

Santisteban, D. A., Mena, M. P., & Abalo, C. (2013). Bridging diversity and family systems: Culturally informed and flexible family-based treatment for Hispanic adolescents. *Couple and Family Psychology: Research and Practice, 2*(4), 246–263.

Santisteban, D. A., Mena, M. P., Gattamorta, K., Gutierrez, M., & Lazarus, R. A. (2024). *Efficacy of a computer assisted and culturally informed family therapy for self-harm behavior in Latine adolescents.* Unpublished manuscript.

Santisteban, D. A., Mena, M. P., & McCabe, B. E. (2011). Preliminary results

for an adaptive family treatment for drug abuse in Hispanic youth. *Journal of Family Psychology, 25*(4), 610–614.
Santisteban, D. A., Mena, M. P., McCabe, B. E., Abalo, C., & Puccinelli, M. (2022). Comparing an individually-based and culturally informed family-based treatment for internalizing, externalizing, and family symptoms in Latino youth. *Family Process., 61*(3), 1144–1161.
Santisteban, D. A., Mena, M. P., Muir, J., McCabe, B. E., Abalo, C., & Cummings, A. M. (2015). The efficacy of two adolescent substance abuse treatments and the impact of comorbid depression: Results of a small randomized controlled trial. *Psychiatric Rehabilitation Journal, 38*(1), 55–64.
Santisteban, D. A., & Szapocznik, J. (1994). Bridging theory, research, and practice to more successfully engage substance abusing youth and their families into therapy. *Journal of Child and Adolescent Substance Abuse, 3*(2), 9–24.
Santisteban, D. A., Szapocznik, J., Perez-Vidal, A., Kurtines, W. M., Murray, E. J., & LaPerriere, A. (1996). Efficacy of intervention for engaging youth and families into treatment and some variables that may contribute to differential effectiveness. *Journal of Family Psychology, 10*(1), 35–44.
Santisteban, D., Vega, R. R., & Suarez-Morales, L. (2006). Utilizing dissemination findings to help understand and bridge the research and practice gap in the treatment of substance abuse disorders in Hispanic populations. *Drug and Alcohol Dependence, 84*(Suppl.), S94-S101.
Schwartz, S. J., & Unger, J. B. (2010). Biculturalism and context: What is biculturalism, and when is it adaptive? *Human Development, 53*(1), 26–32.
Schwartz, S. J., Unger, J. B., Des Rosiers, S. E., Lorenzo-Blanco, E. I., Zamboanga, B. L., Huang, S., . . . Szapocznik, J. (2014). Domains of acculturation and their effects on substance use and sexual behavior in recent Hispanic immigrant adolescents. *Prevention Science, 15*(3), 385–396.
Simpson, D. D. (2002). A conceptual framework for transferring research to practice. *Journal of Substance Abuse Treatment, 22*(4) 171–182.
Sluzki, C. E. (1979). Migration and family conflict. *Family Process, 18*(4), 379–390.
Soto, A., Smith, T. B., Griner, D., Domenech Rodríguez, M. M., & Bernal, G. (2018). Cultural adaptations and therapist multicultural competence: Two meta-analytic reviews. *Journal of Clinical Psychology, 74*(11), 1907–1923.
Stirman, S. W., Kimberly, J., Cook, N., Calloway, A., Castro, F., & Charns, M. (2012). The sustainability of new programs and innovations: A review of the empirical literature and recommendations for future research. *Implementation Science, 7,* 17.
Suárez-Orozco, C., Hee Jin Bang, & Onaga, M. (2010). Contributions to variations in academic trajectories amongst recent immigrant youth. *International Journal of Behavioral Development, 34*(6), 500–510.
Suárez-Orozco, C., & Suárez-Orozco, M. M. (2001). *Children of immigration.* Harvard University Press.
Szapocznik, J., & Kurtines, W. (1989). *Breakthroughs in family therapy with drug abusing and problem youth.* Springer.

Szapocznik, J., Perez-Vidal, A., Brickman, A., Foote, F. H., Santisteban, D., Hervis, O. E., & Kurtines, W. M. (1988). Engaging adolescent drug abusers and their families into treatment: A strategic structural systems approach. *Journal of Consulting and Clinical Psychology, 56*(4), 552–557. (Reprinted in *Annual Review of Addictions Research and Treatment,* 1991, *1,* 331–336.)

Szapocznik, J., Prado, G., Burlew, A. K., Williams, R. A., & Santisteban, D. A. (2007). Drug abuse in African American and Hispanic adolescents: Culture, development, and behavior. *Annual Review of Clinical Psychology, 3*(1), 77–105.

Szapocznik, J., Schwartz, S. J., Muir, J. A., & Brown, C. H. (2012). Brief strategic family therapy: An intervention to reduce adolescent risk behavior. *Couple and Family Psychology, 1*(2), 134–145.

Szapocznik, J., Scopetta, M. A., Aranalde, M. A., & Kurtines, W. M. (1978). Cuban value structure: Clinical implications. *Journal of Consulting and Clinical Psychology, 46*(5), 961–970.

Tudge, J. R., Mokrova, I., Hatfield, B. E., & Karnik, R. B. (2009). Uses and misuses of Bronfenbrenner's bioecological theory of human development. *Journal of Family Theory and Review, 1*(4), 198–210.

Umaña-Taylor, A. J, Quintana, S. M., Lee, R. M., Cross, W. E., Jr., Rivas-Drake, D., Schwartz, S. J., . . . Seaton, E. (2014). Ethnic and racial identity during adolescence and into young adulthood: An integrated conceptualization. *Child Development, 85*(1), 21–39.

Unger, J. B., Schwth, C. J, Fosco, G. M., Lee, Y., & Chen, I.-C. (2016). A component-centered meta-analysis of family-based prevention programs for adolescent substance use. *Clinical Psychology Review, 45,* 72–80.

Vega, W. A., & Gil, A. G. (1998). *Drug use and ethnicity in early adolescence.* SAGE.

Vermeulen-Smit, E., Verduartz, S. J., Huh, J., Soto, D. W., & Baezconde-Garbanati, L. (2014). Acculturation and perceived discrimination: Predictors of substance use trajectories from adolescence to emerging adulthood among Hispanics. *Addictive Behavior, 39*(9), 1293–1296.

U.S. Department of Health and Human Services. (2001). *Mental health: Culture, race and ethnicity—A supplement to Mental health: A report of the Surgeon General.* Author.

Van Ryzin, M. J, Rosermen, J. E., & Engels, R. C. (2015). The effectiveness of family interventions in preventing adolescent illicit drug use: A systematic review and meta-analysis of randomized controlled Trials. *Clinical Child and Family Psychology Review, 18*(3), 218–239.

Wadsworth, T., Kubrin, C. E., & Herting, J. R. (2014). Investigating the rise (and fall) of young Black male suicide in the United States, 1982–2011. *Journal of African American Studies, 18,* 72–91.

Walsh, F. (2016) *Strengthening family resilience* (3rd ed.). Guilford Press.

Watson, M. F. (2019). Facing the Black shadow: Power from the inside out. In M. McGoldrick & K. V. Hardy (Eds.), *Re-visioning family therapy:*

Addressing diversity in clinical practice (3rd ed., pp. 200–214). Guilford Press.

Wilcox, M. M. (2023). Oppression is not "culture": The need to center systemic and structural determinants to address anti-Black racism and racial trauma in psychotherapy. *Psychotherapy, 60*(1), 76.

Yasui, M., & Dishion, T. J. (2007). The ethnic context of child and adolescent problem behavior: Implications for child and family interventions. *Clinical Child and Family Psychology Review, 10*(2), 137–179.

Zayas, L. H., & Gulbas, L. E. (2012). Are suicide attempts by young Latinas a cultural idiom of distress? *Transcultural Psychiatry, 49*(5), 718–734.

Zimbardo, P. G., & Boyd, J. N. (1999). Putting time in perspective: A valid, reliable individual-difference metric. *Journal of Personality and Social Psychology, 27,* 1271–1288.

Index

Note. f or *t* following a page number indicates a figure or table.

ABC Please skill, 142
Acceptance
   adolescent therapy and, 45
   families of LGBTQ+ youth and, 130–132
   familism *(familismo)* and, 42–43
   Motivational Interviewing (MI) strategies and, 45
   psychoeducation and, 10
   Values Orientation Theory and, 41
Acculturation gaps or discrepancies, 129, 134, 166–173
Acculturation module, 69, 143–144, 170, 171. *See also* Acculturation-related experiences; Module material
Acculturation stresses. *See also* Acculturation module; Acculturation-related experiences
   assessment of acculturation and stress, 30–35, 33t, 34t, 35t
   modules focused on, 143–144
   overview, x, 26–27
   tailoring treatment to the individual and, 76–77
Acculturation-related experiences. *See also* Acculturation module; Acculturation stresses; Immigration contexts
   acculturation paradox, 25
   case examples illustrating, 166–173
   Clinical Interview and, 78

family therapy and, 129, 134
   Haitian youth and families and, 212–215
   identifying themes to work on with the adolescent, 92
   integration of cultural themes, 13
   modules focused on, 143–144
   overview, xi, 23–27
   psychoeducation and, 10
   resilience and, 28–30
   tailoring treatment to the individual and, 76–77
Action stage of change, 46, 93. *See also* Change
Activity settings, 50, 51–52
Adaptive approach, 13–14, 106–107
Adaptive interactions, 127–129. *See also* Family interactions
Adolescent developmental stage, 87–89, 103–104, 145–146. *See also* Developmental factors
Adolescent therapy. *See also* Culturally Informed and Flexible Family-Based Treatment for Adolescents (CIFFTA); Psychoeducation
   adolescent developmental stage, 87–89
   Brief Strategic Family Therapy (BSFT), 53–54
   case examples illustrating, 166, 173, 176, 179–180, 186–187
   confidentiality and, 104

239

Adolescent therapy (cont.)
  Ecological Model, 49–52
  engaging and joining the adolescent and, 89–91
  enhancing adolescent motivation, 92–96
  generalizing module material, 99–100
  goals and phases of treatment and, 80t
  identifying themes to work on and, 91–92
  Multidimensional Ecosystemic Comparative Approach (MECA), 55
  overview, 8–10, 43–49, 86–87, 89–105
  preparing for CIFFTA implementation and, 66
  processing of key themes, 96–99
  providing both family and individual therapy and, 83–85, 86–87
  staying on track, 104–105
  Structural Family Therapy, 52–53
  synergy among treatment components and, 10–11, 71
  variability within developmental stages and, 103–104
Adolescents, 116, 137–140, 155. See also Adolescent therapy; Client experiences
Advocacy, family, 148–150
Affirmations, 95. See also Motivational Interviewing (MI) strategies
African American youth and families, 215–219
Aggressive behavior, 109. See also Behavioral problems
Alcohol and Other Substance Use module, 139, 151, 153–154, 183–184, 186. See also Module material
Alcohol misuse, 139. See also Substance misuse
Americanism, 31, 167–168
Assessment. See also Clinical Interview
  of acculturation and stress, 30–35, 33t, 34t, 35t
  case examples illustrating, 160–161, 174, 181, 183
  home-based family therapy, 82
  implementing psychoeducation and, 150
  reluctant family members, 116–117
  of resilience/protective factors, 35–36
  tailoring treatment to the individual and, 73, 74, 75–76

Assimilation, 24, 166–173. See also Acculturation-related experiences
Asylum seekers, xvi. See also Immigration contexts
Attention-Deficit/Hyperactivity Disorder module, 137–138. See also Module material
Autonomy, 5, 9, 88, 94

B

Behavioral problems. See also Risk-taking behavior; Triggers of behavior
  adolescent therapy and, 43–44, 91–92, 101–103
  case examples illustrating, 166–173
  DBT skills training and, 47–48
  overview, x
  systemic conceptualization and, 108–109
Bias, 46–47
Bicultural profiles, 24, 167–168. See also Acculturation-related experiences
Biopsychosocial processes, 51
Black youth and families, 215–219
Blaming interactions, 124–125. See also Family interactions
Blended Family module, 147–148. See also Module material; Parenting modules
Blocking, 123–124
Bond between therapist and client, 55. See also Therapeutic relationship
Borderline personality disorder profile, 47–48
Brief Strategic Family Therapy (BSFT), 53–54, 86

C

Change
  enhancing adolescent motivation and, 92–96
  family therapy and, 114–116
  goals and phases of treatment and, 80t
  motivation enhancement and, 44–45
  Motivational Interviewing (MI) strategies and, 45–46
  psychoeducation and, 158

Structural Family Therapy and, 52–53
tailoring treatment to the individual and, 74
CIFFTA (Culturally Informed and Flexible Family-Based Treatment for Adolescents). *See* Culturally Informed and Flexible Family-Based Treatment for Adolescents (CIFFTA)
CIFFTA Clinical Interview. *See* Clinical Interview
CIFFTA Postsession Therapist Self-Report of Adherence. *See* Postsession Therapist Self-Report of Adherence
CIFFTA Tailoring Report. *See* Tailoring Report
CIFFTA Treatment Plan. *See* Treatment Plan
Client experiences. *See also* Cultural contexts; Immigration contexts; Latine youth and families
acculturation-related experiences, 23–27
assessment of acculturation and stress and, 30–35, 33*t*, 34*t*, 35*t*
assessment of resilience/protective factors and, 35–36
minority stress and, 27–28
overview, 20–21, 36–37
parent–child separations and, 21–23
reception in the host country and, 28
resilience and, 28–30
Clinical Interview. *See also* Assessment
case examples illustrating, 160–161, 174, 176, 181
implementing psychoeducation and, 150
preparing for CIFFTA implementation and, 67
tailoring treatment to the individual and, 73, 77–79
Coerced adolescents or families, 111–112. *See also* Juvenile justice system
Coercive Family Processes, 107. *See also* Family interactions
Collaborative approach. *See also* Therapists
case examples illustrating, 163, 176
challenges to implementing CIFFTA's psychoeducational component and, 156–157
enhancing adolescent motivation and, 94

overview, 70
psychoeducation and, 152
Communication skills. *See also* Interpersonal effectiveness
adolescent therapy and, 100, 101
case examples illustrating, 166–173
reducing conflictual and hostile interactions and, 122–127
shaping more adaptive and supportive relationship interactions, 127–129
Community partnerships, 219–220
Community treatment agencies, 202–207
Competencies, 5, 192–193, 195. *See also* Therapists
Conduct problems, 9, 180–187. *See also* Behavioral problems
Confidentiality, 84–85, 90, 104
Conflict, family. *See* Family interactions
Conflict in therapy sessions, 112, 122–129, 134. *See also* Family interactions
Contemplation stage of change, 46, 93. *See also* Change
Contextual framework, 49–52
Couple subsystem, 117, 132
CRAFFT (Car, Relax, Alone, Forget, Friends, Trouble), 74
Crisis management, 48, 219–220
Crisis Survival Skills, 143
Cultural contexts. *See also* Client experiences
Clinical Interview and, 77
cultural competencies and, 5
culture-related stressors, 143–145, 159–173, 174–175, 181–182
families of LGBTQ+ youth and, 130
family therapy and, 114, 129, 130
identity formation and, 46–47
integration of cultural themes, 11–13
modules focused on, 143–145
Multidimensional Ecosystemic Comparative Approach (MECA), 55
overview, xi–xii, 6, 38–43
Cultural Formulation Interview (CFI), 34
Culturally centered treatments, 4–5
Culturally Informed and Flexible Family-Based Treatment for Adolescents (CIFFTA). *See also* Adolescent therapy; Family therapy; Individual therapy; Module material; Psychoeducation; Therapists; Training
adaptive and flexible framework of, 13–14

CIFFTA (cont.)
  community partners and, 219–220
  efficacy and effectiveness of, 15–19
  extending to non-Latine populations, 211–219
  future directions, 220–222
  individual therapy component of, 8–10, 83–85
  integration of cultural themes into, 11–13
  online training and, 195–207
  overview, ix, xvii–xviii, 6–19, 38, 55–56, 59, 85, 135–136, 220–222
  pillars of, 49–55
  providing both family and individual therapy and, 83–85
  psychoeducational component of, 10, 150–158
  synergy between treatment components, 10–11

D

Dating, 145, 150
Delivery of CIFFTA, 79, 81–85. *See also* Implementation of CIFFTA
Depression, 137, 159–166, 174–187. *See also* Depression module
Depression module, 69, 137, 150, 164–165. *See also* Module material
Developmental factors
  adolescent developmental stage, 87–89, 103–104, 145–146
  identifying themes to work on with the adolescent, 91
  modules focused on, 145–146
  tailoring treatment to the individual and, 74
  variability within, 103–104
Diagnostic and Statistical Manual of Mental Disorders (DSM-IV-TR), 15, 34
Dialectical Behavioral Therapy (DBT), 47–49, 83, 142
Diary cards, 102, 180
Directive stance of therapist, 64–65. *See also* Therapists
Discrimination. *See also* Discrimination module
  acculturation-related experiences and, 24, 26
  adolescent therapy and, 96, 97, 99
  Black youth and families and, 215–219
  identifying themes to work on with the adolescent, 92
  psychoeducation and, 10
  systemic conceptualization and, 107
  therapists and, 210
  training and, 62
Discrimination module, 145, 183, 184, 186, 187. *See also* Module material
Distal stressors, 28, 97–98, 210
Distress tolerance, 48, 143. *See also* Distress Tolerance module
Distress Tolerance module, 143, 176, 177, 179. *See also* Module material
Diversion programs, 89–90, 180–187, 211. *See also* Juvenile justice system

E

Early adolescence, 87, 103–104. *See also* Adolescent developmental stage
Ecological context, 39, 49–52, 55, 213
Effectiveness of CIFFTA, 15–19, 85. *See also* Implementation of CIFFTA
Emerging adulthood, 87, 103–104. *See also* Adolescent developmental stage
Emotion Regulation module, 142, 150, 151, 170, 171–172, 173, 176, 177, 179, 183, 184, 187. *See also* Module material
Emotion regulation skills. *See also* Emotion Regulation module
  adolescent therapy and, 100
  DBT skills training and, 48
  distress tolerance and, 143
  individual therapy and, 8
  reducing conflictual and hostile interactions and, 125
  skills development modules and, 142
  systemic conceptualization and, 109
Enactments, 122–123
Engagement
  adolescent therapy and, 89–91
  Black youth and families and, 217–218
  Brief Strategic Family Therapy (BSFT), 54
  case examples illustrating, 162–163, 169–170, 175–176, 182–184
  Clinical Interview and, 77
  families of LGBTQ+ youth and, 130
  family therapy and, 110–119, 130, 134

goals and phases of treatment and, 80t
initiator of therapy keeping another
  caregiver out of therapy, 118–119
motivation enhancement and, 44–46
reluctant family members and, 116–118
training and, 195
virtual delivery of CIFFTA and, 81–82
Ethnic identity, 9, 46–47, 98–99, 215–
  219. *See also* Identity formation
Evidence-based treatments (EBTs).
  See also Culturally Informed and
  Flexible Family-Based Treatment for
  Adolescents (CIFFTA)
  community treatment agencies and,
    202–207
  efficacy and effectiveness of CIFFTA
    and, 18
  overview, ix–xi, 4–5, 6, 19, 38,
    191–192, 207–208
  training and, 61, 192–193
Experiences, client. *See* Client experiences
Expert stance, 156–157. *See also*
  Therapists

F

Familism (*familismo*). *See also* Family
  processes
  full family involvement and, 113
  integration of cultural themes, 12
  overview, 29–30, 42–43
  Values Orientation Theory and, 39
Family advocacy, 148–150
Family history, 75–76, 77
Family interactions. *See also*
  Communication skills; Family
  processes; Family therapy;
  Interpersonal effectiveness; Parenting
  practices
  adolescent therapy and, 96, 101
  blocking and, 123–124
  case examples illustrating, 166–173,
    174, 180–187
  changing the interaction sequence,
    125–127
  generalizing information and skills and,
    120–122, 153–154
  goals and phases of treatment and, 80t
  identifying processes and interactions,
    119–120
  overview, 107, 146–150

reducing conflictual and hostile
  interactions, 122–127
reframing and, 124–125
shaping more adaptive and supportive
  relationship interactions, 127–129,
  134
tailoring treatment to the individual
  and, 75–76
training and, 195
Family involvement. *See also* Engagement;
  Family interactions; Family therapy
  choosing who will receive the modules
    and, 150–151
  full family involvement, 112–114
  initiator of therapy keeping another
    caregiver out of therapy, 118–119
  reluctant family members, 116–118
Family life cycle, 55, 75–76, 132–133, 134
Family processes. *See also* Familism
  (*familismo*); Family interactions
  Clinical Interview and, 77–78
  full family involvement and, 112–114
  generalizing information and skills
    and, 153–154
  Haitian youth and families and,
    212–213
  identifying processes and interactions,
    119–120
  identity formation and, 47
  impact of racism and, 216–219
  Multidimensional Ecosystemic
    Comparative Approach (MECA), 55
  overview, 5–6, 7–8, 42, 59–60
  reducing conflictual and hostile
    interactions and, 122–127
  tailoring treatment to the individual
    and, 75
Family resilience. *See* Resilience
Family therapy. *See also* Culturally
  Informed and Flexible Family-Based
  Treatment for Adolescents (CIFFTA);
  Psychoeducation
  Black youth and families and, 217–218
  Brief Strategic Family Therapy (BSFT),
    53–54
  case examples illustrating, 165–166,
    172–173, 178–179, 184–186
  engagement and joining the family and,
    107, 110–119
  families of LGBTQ+ youth, 130–132
  family life cycle stages, 132–133
  family processes and, 107

244 ■ Index

Family therapy (cont.)
  full family involvement, 112–114
  generalizing information and skills, 120–122
  goals and phases of treatment and, 80t
  home-based family therapy, 82–83
  identifying processes and interactions, 119–120
  overview, 3–4, 10–11, 59–60, 106–107, 134, 221–222
  preparing for CIFFTA implementation and, 65–79, 65t, 68f
  providing both family and individual therapy and, 83–85, 86–87
  psychoeducation and, 158
  reducing conflictual and hostile interactions, 122–127
  shaping more adaptive and supportive relationship interactions, 127–129
  staying on track, 133–134
  Structural Family Therapy and, 52–53
  synergy among treatment components and, 71
  systemic conceptualization and, 107, 108–109
  variability within developmental stages and, 103–104
  virtual delivery of, 81–82
  working with key subsystems and, 132–133
Flexibility, 13–14, 106–107

G

Gender identity. *See also* Gender Identity and Sexual Orientation module; Identity formation; LGBTQ+ youth; Sexual orientation
  family therapy and, 130–132
  individual therapy and, 8, 9, 96–98
  overview, 141
  terminology, xiv
Gender Identity and Sexual Orientation module, 141, 176, 177–178, 179–180. *See also* Module material
Generalized Anxiety Disorder–7 (GAD-7), 73
Generalizing skills
  adolescent therapy and, 99–100
  case examples illustrating, 165–166, 172–173, 178–180

family therapy and, 120–122
module material and, 136, 153–154, 158
overview, 136, 153–154
synergy between CIFFTA's components and, 10–11
Goal setting, 8, 9, 173
Goals of treatment, 55, 78–79, 80t

H

Haitian youth and families, 211–215
Health Promotion module, 138, 150. *See also* Module material
Hispanic Family Resilience Measure (HFRM), 35–36
Hispanic Optimism Psychological Examination (HOPE), 35–36
Hispanic Stress Inventory–2 (HSI-2), 30–31, 33–35, 34t, 35t, 76, 167
Hispanic Stress Inventory—Adolescent Version (HSI-A), 30–31, 32–33, 33t, 35
Hispanicism, 167–168
Home-based family therapy, 82–83. *See also* Family therapy
Hope/hopelessness, 114–116, 140
Hospitalization, 219–220
Hostile interactions, 122–127. *See also* Family interactions

I

Identity formation. *See also* Cultural contexts; Gender identity; Racial identity
  adolescent developmental stage and, 87–89
  adolescent therapy and, 46–47, 96–99
  family therapy and, 129, 130–132
  identifying themes to work on with the adolescent, 92
Immigration contexts. *See also* Client experiences
  acculturation-related experiences, 23–27
  assessment of acculturation and stress, 30–35, 33t, 34t, 35t
  case examples illustrating, 159–173
  Clinical Interview and, 78

ecological systems theory and, 50
evolving perspectives on, xii–xiii
Haitian youth and families and, 211
identity formation and, 47
integration of cultural themes, 13
minority stress and, 27–28
modules focused on, 143–145
overview, x, xi
parent–child separations and, 21–23
reasons for migration to the United States, xv
reception in the host country and, 28
resilience and, 28–30
synergy among treatment components and, 72
types of immigrants, xv–xvii
Immigration-Related Separation module, 144, 150. *See also* Module material; Parent–child separations; Separation module
Implementation of CIFFTA. *See also* Adolescent therapy; Culturally Informed and Flexible Family-Based Treatment for Adolescents (CIFFTA); Family therapy; Individual therapy
community treatment agencies and, 202–207
decisions regarding, 79, 81–85
improving, 207
overview, 85, 208
preparing for, 65–79, 65t, 68f
psychoeducation and, 150–158
staying on track and, 104–105, 133–134, 157–158
synergy among treatment components and, 70–72
tailoring treatment to the individual and, 73–79
training and, 61–65, 63f
Individual experiences. *See* Client experiences
Individual therapy. *See* Adolescent therapy; Culturally Informed and Flexible Family-Based Treatment for Adolescents (CIFFTA)
Internalized homophobia, 97–98
Interpersonal effectiveness. *See also* Communication skills; Family interactions; Interpersonal Effectiveness module
adolescent therapy and, 100, 101
DBT skills training and, 48
generalizing information and skills and, 153–154
identifying themes to work on with the adolescent, 92
individual therapy and, 8, 9
skills development modules and, 142–143
Interpersonal Effectiveness module, 142–143, 150, 151, 170, 171–172, 173, 183, 184, 187. *See also* Module material
Interpersonal violence, 50, 145, 150, 212

J

Joining
adolescent therapy and, 89–91
case examples illustrating, 162–163, 169–170, 175–176, 182–184
family therapy and, 110–119
Just-in-time (JIT) learning and support framework, 194. *See also* Training
Juvenile justice system. *See also* Legal context
case examples illustrating, 180–187
engaging and joining the adolescent and, 89–90
family therapy and, 111–112
Haitian youth and families and, 211
modules focused on, 148–149
overview, 56
tailoring treatment to the individual and, 74

K

Key themes, 96–100

L

Language, 129, 213
Late adolescence/young adulthood, 87, 103–104. *See also* Adolescent developmental stage
Latine youth and families, x, xiii–xv, 4–5, 20–21. *See also* Client experiences
Legal context. *See also* Juvenile justice system; Legal System module
case examples illustrating, 180–187
engaging and joining the adolescent and, 89–90

Legal context (*cont.*)
  family interactions and, 101
  modules focused on, 148–149
  overview, x, 56
  psychoeducation and, 10
  tailoring treatment to the individual and, 74
Legal System module, 148–149. *See also* Module material
LGBTQ+ youth. *See also* Gender identity; Gender Identity and Sexual Orientation module; Sexual orientation
  adolescent therapy and, 8, 9, 96–98
  case examples illustrating, 174–180
  familism (*familismo*) and, 42–43
  family therapy and, 130–132, 134
  integration of cultural themes, 13
  minority stress and, 28
  modules focused on, 141
  psychoeducation and, 10
Life cycle, family, 55, 75–76, 132–133, 134
Life skills, 9, 92. *See also* Psychoeducation; Skills training

M

Macrosystem, 50
Maintenance, 80*t*, 103
Maintenance stage of change, 46, 93. *See also* Change
Marginalization, 26, 56, 92, 97
Marital stress, 76
Mastery of competencies, 192–193, 207–208
Medication module, 149–150. *See also* Module material
Mesosystems, 51
Middle adolescence, 87, 103–104. *See also* Adolescent developmental stage
Migration. *See also* Immigration contexts
  assessment of acculturation and stress and, 34
  case examples illustrating, 159–166
  Clinical Interview and, 78
  Haitian youth and families and, 211–215
  Multidimensional Ecosystemic Comparative Approach (MECA), 55

parent–child separations and, 21–23
reasons for migration to the United States, xv
Mindfulness, 48, 142
Minority stress, 27–28, 97, 210, 217. *See also* Client experiences
Minority Stress Model, 27–28, 97–98, 209–211
Modulation, 48
Module material. *See also* Culturally Informed and Flexible Family-Based Treatment for Adolescents (CIFFTA); Generalizing skills; Psychoeducation; Skills training; *individual modules*
  adolescent therapy and, 99–100
  case examples illustrating, 163–165, 170–172, 176–178, 183–184, 185, 186, 187
  challenges to implementing, 154–157
  choosing when and how to deliver, 151–152
  choosing who will receive the modules and, 150–151
  culture and culture-related stressors, 143–145
  developmental stage, 145–146
  family advocacy in the youth's ecology, 148–150
  family therapy and, 121–122
  gender identity and sexual orientation and, 141
  generalizing information and skills from, 136, 153–154
  implementing psychoeducation and, 150–158
  overview, 66–70, 68*f*, 80*t*, 135–136, 158
  parenting and the family, 146–150
  skills development, 141–143
  staying on track and, 157–158
  youth symptomatology, 137–140
Motivation
  acculturation-related experiences and, 24
  adolescent therapy and, 8, 44–46
  enhancing adolescent motivation, 92–96
  goals and phases of treatment and, 80*t*
  identifying themes to work on with the adolescent, 91

tailoring treatment to the individual and, 74
training and, 195
Motivational Interviewing (MI) strategies
adolescent therapy and, 45–46, 94–96
case examples illustrating, 183
individual therapy and, 9
variability within developmental stages and, 103–104
Multidimensional Ecosystemic Comparative Approach (MECA), 55
Multiple minorities, 28. *See also* Minority stress
Multiple therapists, 83–85. *See also* Therapists

N

Natural Helper and Community Health Worker framework, 219
Negative interactions, 122–127, 134. *See also* Family interactions
Negotiation, 39–40
Nonjudgmental stance, 95, 152

O

OARS (open-ended questions, affirmations, reflections, and summaries), 95. *See also* Motivational Interviewing (MI) strategies
Observation, 107, 119–120
Online delivery, 81–82, 221. *See also* Technology-assisted interventions; Virtual delivery of CIFFTA
Online training, 193–207. *See also* Training
Open-ended questions, 95. *See also* Motivational Interviewing (MI) strategies
Opposite action skill, 142
Organizational culture, 202–207
Overinvolvement, 5, 125–127

P

Parental advocacy, 148–150
Parental subsystem, 132–133

Parent–child separations. *See also* Immigration-Related Separation module; Separation module
case examples illustrating, 159–166
ecological systems theory and, 52
modules focused on, 144
overview, 5, 21–23
synergy among treatment components and, 72
Parenting modules. *See also* Module material
case examples illustrating, 164, 170–171, 176–177, 183, 185
overview, 69, 146–148, 151
synergy among treatment components and, 71
Parenting practices. *See also* Family interactions; Parenting modules
Black youth and families and, 216
case examples illustrating, 164, 165–173
Clinical Interview and, 78
familism (*familismo*) and, 30
Haitian youth and families and, 213
modules focused on, 146–150
parental advocacy and, 148–150
parent–child separations and, 23
providing both family and individual therapy and, 84–85
psychoeducation and, 10
Patient Health Questionnaire–9 (PHQ-9), 73
Peer learning network (PLN), 201–202. *See also* Training
Peer relationships, 92, 186–187
Postsession Therapist Self-Report of Adherence
adolescent therapy and, 104–105
family therapy and, 133–134
psychoeducation and, 157–158
Posttraumatic stress disorder (PTSD), 140. *See also* Traumatic experiences
Power struggles, 44–45
Practices, 24, 195–196
Precontemplation stage of change, 46, 93. *See also* Change
Prejudice. *See* Discrimination; Racism
Preparation stage of change, 46, 93. *See also* Change
Present orientation, 41–42
Presenting problem, 73, 108–109

Previous therapy experiences, 114–116
Problem Behavior Syndrome, 43–44. *See also* Behavioral problems
Protective factors. *See also* Resilience
assessment of, 35–36
case examples illustrating, 167, 174, 181, 185
families of LGBTQ+ youth and, 131
impact of racism and, 216–219
overview, 28–30, 187
tailoring treatment to the individual and, 77
Proximal stressors
adolescent therapy and, 97–98
ecological systems theory and, 49–50, 51–52
overview, 28
therapists and, 210
Psychiatric evaluation, 149–150. *See also* Assessment
Psychoeducation. *See also* Module material; Skills training
case examples illustrating, 163–165, 170–172, 176–178, 183–184, 185, 186, 187
Clinical Interview and, 77
DBT skills training and, 47–48
future directions and, 221
generalizing information and skills from, 136, 153–154
goals and phases of treatment and, 80*t*
Haitian youth and families and, 214
implementing, 66, 150–158
individual therapy and, 9
modules focused on youth symptomatology, 137–140
overview, 10, 135–136, 158
synergy among treatment components and, 10–11, 71, 72
Punishment, therapy as, 111–112, 181–182

R

Racial identity, 9, 46–47, 98–99, 215–219. *See also* Identity formation
Racism
adolescent therapy and, 96, 97, 99
Black youth and families and, 215–219
Haitian youth and families and, 211
resilience and, 29
systemic conceptualization and, 107
training and, 62, 196
Radical Acceptance skills, 143
Rationale for therapy, 112–114
Readiness, 152, 158
Referrals, 83–85, 219–220
Reflections, 95. *See also* Motivational Interviewing (MI) strategies
Reframing, 124–125, 185
Refugees, xvi. *See also* Immigration contexts
Rejection, 130, 174
Relapse prevention, 80*t*, 103
Relapse prevention stage of change, 93
Reluctant clients, 116–118, 174–180. *See also* Legal context; Resistance
Research practice gap, 191–192. *See also* Evidence-based treatments (EBTs)
Research support for CIFFTA, 15–19
Residential treatment, 219–220
Resilience. *See also* Protective factors
assessment of, 35–36
Black youth and families and, 219
families of LGBTQ+ youth and, 131
overview, 28–30
tailoring treatment to the individual and, 77
Resistance
Brief Strategic Family Therapy (BSFT), 54
challenging the label of, 111–112
engaging and joining the adolescent and, 90–91
family therapy and, 111–112
reluctant family members, 116–118
Respeto (respect) value, 39–40
Reunification, 22–23, 159–166. *See also* Parent–child separations
Reverse-classroom framework, 193. *See also* Training
Risk factors, 28–30, 187
Risk-taking behavior, 43–44, 87–89, 101–103, 174–187. *See also* Behavioral problems; Self-harm risk; Sexual behavior; Substance misuse; Triggers of behavior
Risky Sexual Behavior module, 71, 139, 150. *See also* Module material
Role plays, 101, 192–193

S

School context, 149, 159–173, 180–187
School module, 149. *See also* Module material
Screening, 73, 74. *See also* Assessment
Second-culture acquisition. *See* Acculturation-related experiences
Self-Harm module, 69, 72, 138, 177–178, 179–180. *See also* Module material
Self-harm risk. *See also* Risk-taking behavior; Self-Harm module
  adolescent therapy and, 101–103
  case examples illustrating, 174–180
  overview, x, 138
  psychoeducation and, 10
  synergy among treatment components and, 72
Separation. *See* Parent–child separations
Separation module, 164, 165. *See also* Immigration-Related Separation module; Module material; Parent–child separations
Sexual behavior, 13, 74, 139
Sexual orientation. *See also* Gender Identity and Sexual Orientation module; LGBTQ+ youth
  adolescent therapy and, 96–98
  case examples illustrating, 174–180
  family therapy and, 130–132
  individual therapy and, 8, 9
  modules focused on, 141
Shared decision-making process, 67, 158
Sibling subsystem, 133, 185
Single Parenting module, 147, 183. *See also* Module material; Parenting modules
Skills training, 47–49, 80*t*, 141–143. *See also* Module material; Psychoeducation
Social media, 10. *See also* Social Media module
Social Media module, 145–146. *See also* Module material
Social skills. *See* Interpersonal effectiveness; Interpersonal Effectiveness module
Stages of change, 45–46, 92–93. *See also* Change
Standardization of training content, 200–201. *See also* Training
Strengths. *See* Protective factors; Resilience
Stress, 92, 209–210
Structural Family Therapy, 52–53
Structural racism. *See* Racism
Substance misuse. *See also* Substance Use module
  case examples illustrating, 180–187
  conflictual and hostile interactions and, 126–127
  family interactions and, 101
  family work and, 9
  individual therapy and, 8
  overview, x, 139
  psychoeducation and, 10
  synergy among treatment components and, 70–71
  tailoring treatment to the individual and, 74
Substance Use module, 71. *See also* Module material
Subsystems, 132–133, 134
Suicide risk, x, 97, 130, 138
Suicide Risk module, 138. *See also* Module material
Summaries, 95. *See also* Motivational Interviewing (MI) strategies
Supportive interactions, 127–129. *See also* Family interactions
Sustainment, 202–207, 208
Symptoms, 73, 108–109, 137–140
Syndemics, 44
Synergy, 70–72
Systemic conceptualization, 62, 63*f*, 108–109, 134, 195
Systemic perspective, 49–52, 61–62, 63*f*

T

Tailoring Report
  case examples illustrating, 160–161, 163, 167, 174, 176, 181, 183
  identifying themes to work on with the adolescent, 91–92
  implementation of CIFFTA and, 67–69, 68*f*, 150
  synergy among treatment components and, 71
Tailoring training to the individual, 200–201. *See also* Training

Tailoring treatment to the individual adolescent/family, 66–70, 68f. *See also* Tailoring Report
   case examples illustrating, 162–165, 169–172, 175–178, 182–184
   overview, 73–79, 85, 187
   training and, 195
Technology-assisted interventions, 16, 79, 81–82, 221
Teen Dating and Interpersonal Violence module, 145, 150. *See also* Module material
Telehealth. *See* Virtual delivery of CIFFTA
Terminology, x, xiii–xv, xvii
Therapeutic relationship
   Black youth and families and, 217–218
   bond between therapist and client, 55
   case examples illustrating, 163
   engaging and joining the adolescent and, 89–91
   family therapy and, 110
Therapists. *See also* Training
   adolescent therapy and, 83–85, 104–105
   Black youth and families and, 217–218
   community treatment agencies and, 202–207
   cultural competencies and, 5
   delivery of individual and family therapy and, 83–85
   enhancing adolescent motivation and, 95–96
   family interactions and, 127–128
   family therapy and, 83–85, 115–116, 133–134
   implementation of CIFFTA and, 61–65, 63f, 85, 155, 156–157
   modules and, 151–152, 157–158
   reducing conflictual and hostile interactions and, 122
Timeline Followback interview, 74
Traditionalism-modernism continuum, 43
Training. *See also* Therapists
   case examples illustrating, 196–198
   community treatment agencies and, 202–207
   implementation of CIFFTA and, 61–65, 63f, 85
   improving, 207
   online platform for, 135, 193–207
   overview, 192–193, 207–208, 210
   racial sensitivity and, 218

Training and Implementation Associates (TIA), 195
Transdiagnostic approach, 14, 69–70
Transgender youth. *See* Gender identity; LGBTQ+ youth
Transparency, 84
Trauma module, 139–140. *See also* Module material
Trauma-Focused Cognitive Behavioral Therapy (TF-CBT), 106
Traumatic experiences, 34, 50, 92, 139–140
Treatment delivery, 79, 81–85. *See also* Implementation of CIFFTA
Treatment Plan
   adolescent therapy and, 104–105
   family therapy and, 133–134
   psychoeducation and, 157–158
Treatment planning, 82. *See also* Treatment Plan
Treatment processes, 38–43, 55–56
Treatment-seeking behavior, 38–43
Triggers of behavior, 101–103, 109, 125–126, 186–187. *See also* Behavioral problems; Risk-taking behavior
Trust, 90, 131, 217–218

V

Values, 24, 38–43, 214. *See also* Familism (*familismo*)
Values Orientation Theory, 38, 39–42
Virtual delivery of CIFFTA, 81–82, 221. *See also* Technology-assisted interventions
Voluntary immigrants, xvi. *See also* Immigration contexts

W

Wise Mind ACCEPTS skills, 143
Worldviews
   cultural contexts and, 38–43
   families of LGBTQ+ youth and, 130
   family therapy and, 114, 129, 130
   Haitian youth and families and, 214

Y

Young adulthood, 87, 103–104. *See also* Adolescent developmental stage